# ADULT HEALTH AND HUMAN CAPITAL

# ADULT HEALTH AND HUMAN CAPITAL

## Impact of Birth Weight and Childhood Growth

## SANTOSH K. BHARGAVA

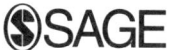

Los Angeles | London | New Delhi
Singapore | Washington DC | Melbourne

*First published in 2018 by*

 **SAGE Publications India Pvt Ltd**
B1/I-1 Mohan Cooperative Industrial Area
Mathura Road, New Delhi 110 044, India
*www.sagepub.in*

**SAGE Publications Inc**
2455 Teller Road
Thousand Oaks, California 91320, USA

**SAGE Publications Ltd**
1 Oliver's Yard, 55 City Road
London EC1Y 1SP, United Kingdom

**SAGE Publications Asia-Pacific Pte Ltd**
3 Church Street
#10-04 Samsung Hub
Singapore 049483

Published by Vivek Mehra for SAGE Publications India Pvt Ltd, typeset in 10/12 pts Times New Roman by Zaza Eunice, Hosur, Tamil Nadu, India and printed at Chaman Enterprises, New Delhi.

**Library of Congress Cataloging-in-Publication Data**

Name: Bhargava, Santosh K., author.
Title: Adult health & human capital: impact of birth weight and childhood
    growth/Santosh K. Bhargava.
Other titles: Adult health and human capital
Description: New Delhi; Thousand Oaks, California: SAGE Publications India
    Pvt Ltd, 2017. | Includes bibliographical references and index.
Identifiers: LCCN 2017023293| ISBN 9789386446855 (print hb: alk. paper) |
    ISBN 9789386446879 (e pub 2.0) | ISBN 9789386446862 (e book)
Subjects: | MESH: Growth and Development | Birth Weight | Infant | Child |
    Cohort Studies | Health Status | Diet–adverse effects | Chronic
    Disease–epidemiology | India–epidemiology
Classification: LCC RA792 | NLM WS 103 | DDC 614.4/2–dc23 LC record available at https://lccn.
loc.gov/2017023293

**ISBN:** 978-93-864-4685-5 (HB)

**SAGE Team:** Rajesh Dey, Guneet Kaur Gulati, Shobana Paul and Ritu Chopra

*Dedicated to*
*my wife Manorama, who made me what I am, and to*
*my wonderful children, who supported me all the way*

Thank you for choosing a SAGE product!
If you have any comment, observation or feedback,
I would like to personally hear from you.

*Please write to me at* **contactceo@sagepub.in**

**Vivek Mehra,** Managing Director and CEO, SAGE India.

## Bulk Sales

SAGE India offers special discounts
for purchase of books in bulk.
We also make available special imprints
and excerpts from our books on demand.

*For orders and enquiries, write to us at*

Marketing Department
SAGE Publications India Pvt Ltd
B1/I-1, Mohan Cooperative Industrial Area
Mathura Road, Post Bag 7
New Delhi 110044, India

*E-mail us at* **marketing@sagepub.in**

### Get to know more about SAGE

Be invited to SAGE events, get on our mailing list.
*Write today to* **marketing@sagepub.in**

This book is also available as an e-book.

# Contents

| | |
|---|---:|
| *List of Tables* | ix |
| *List of Figures* | xiii |
| *List of Abbreviations* | xvii |
| *Foreword* by K. Srinath Reddy | xix |
| *Preface* | xxi |
| *Acknowledgements* | xxv |
| **Introduction** | 1 |
| **Part 1  Background of the Study** | 5 |
| 1  Genesis | 7 |
| 2  Launching of the Study | 24 |
| 3  Demography | 29 |
| **Part 2  The Cohort** | 47 |
| 1  Pregnancy | 49 |
| 2  Birth and Outcome of Cohort | 53 |
| 3  Low Birth Weight | 67 |
| 4  Child Survival, Health, and Disease | 93 |
| **Part 3  Growth, Cognitive Development, and Nutrition** | 101 |
| 1  Growth | 103 |
| 2  Cognitive Development | 120 |
| 3  Nutrition | 129 |
| **Part 4  Transition to Adult Phase** | 137 |
| 1  Assembling the Cohort | 139 |
| 2  The Beginning of the Adult Period | 143 |
| 3  Re-establishing the New Delhi Birth Cohort | 148 |
| 4  Environments, Social and Cultural Changes | 156 |

**Part 5   Childhood Growth, Adult Health, and Human Capital**   163
   1  Body Growth, Adult Health, and Disease   165
   2  Size at Birth, BMI, Body Composition, and Chronic
      Adult Diseases   173
   3  Body Growth and Human Capital Development   179
   4  Parental Influences on Adult Health   182
   5  Body Growth, Genetic Studies, and Adult Health
      Outcome   185

**Part 6   Intergenerational and Trans-generational Studies**   189
   1  The Intergenerational Change in F1 and F2 Generation   193
   2  The Third Generation   204

**Part 7   Community Expectations and Challenges**   209
   1  Attrition or Loss to Follow-Up   211
   2  Cohort Participation   218

**Part 8   Implications and Impact**   225
   1  Public Health and Policies   228
   2  The NDBC Research   231
   3  Childhood Growth, Adult Health, and Human Capital   237
   4  Intergeneration and Trans-generational Changes   242
   5  Challenges to Community Participation   245

**Part 9   Summation**   247

*Appendix*   263
*Bibliography*   271
*Index*   279
*About the Author*   286

# List of Tables

1.3.1    Area-wise Per Capita Income    30

1.3.2    Mean Age at Marriage by Per Capita Income and Literacy    36

2.1.1    Profile of Pregnant Women    51

2.2.1    Gestation Distribution from 30 Weeks to 42+ Weeks in Cohort Subjects    56

2.2.2    Factors Influencing Gestational Age in Cohort Subjects    57

2.2.3    Birth Measurements Mean Weight, Length, and Head Circumference in Both Sexes in Cohort Subjects    60

2.2.4    Mean Birth Weight, Length, and Head Circumference at Different Gestation Period in Cohort Subjects    63

2.3.1    Causes of LBW in Cohort Subjects    72

2.3.2    Mortality Pattern and Intrauterine Growth in Cohort Subjects    76

2.3.3    Mean Length/Height (cm) Comparison in Birth Weight $< 2,500 \, g$ (LBW) and Birth Weight $\geq 2,500 \, g$ (Normal) in Cohort Subjects from Birth to 20 Years at Different Age Periods    77

2.3.4    Mean Weight (kg) Comparison in Birth Weight $< 2,500 \, g$ (LBW) and Birth Weight $\geq 2,500$ g (Normal) in Cohort Subjects from Birth to 20 Years at Different Age Periods    77

2.3.5    Mean Weight (kg) for Different Categories of Birth Weight in Cohort Subjects at Different Age Periods    78

2.3.6    Mean Length/Height (cm) for Different Categories of Birth Weight in Cohort Subjects at Different Age Periods    78

2.3.7    Preterm and Term Weight and Height Growth Pattern in Cohort Subjects    81

2.3.8    Mean Comparison of Length/Height at Different Ages Among the Categories of Foetal Centiles for Length in the Cohort Subjects    83

2.3.9    Mean Comparison of Weight at Different Ages Among the Categories of Foetal Centiles for Weight in the Cohort Subjects   83

2.3.10   Intellectual Development and Mother's Socio-economic Status in LBW and Normal Cohort Subjects   86

2.3.11   Intellectual Development and Mother's Educational Status in LBW and Normal Cohort Subjects   87

2.3.12   Mean IQ Levels on LBW and Normal Cohort Subjects at 5–6 Years of Age   88

2.3.13   Intellectual Development in LBW and Normal Cohort Subjects at 5–6 Years of Age   88

2.3.14   Mean IQ Levels in Preterm, AGA, Term, Small for Gestation, and Cohort Subjects at 5–6 Years of Age   88

2.3.15   Life Course of LBW in Cohort Subjects   90

2.4.1    Mortality Among Cohort Subjects from 0–5 Years of Age   95

2.4.2    Perinatal and Under-five Mortality in Cohort Subjects with Birth Weight < 2,500 g (LBW) and $\geq 2,500$ g   98

3.1.1    Body Growth in Weight from Birth to 20 Years in Cohort Subjects   109

3.1.2    Mean WHO Anthropometric Z Scores from Birth to 20 Years Age of Cohorts   117

3.2.1    Mean IQ and CD Score of 4 Years Old Cohort Subjects   123

3.2.2    CD Scores of 6 Years Old Cohort Subjects   125

3.3.1    Distribution by $Z < -2$ in the Cohort Subjects by Gender at Different Ages for Stunting, Underweight, and Wasting   132

3.3.2    Prevalence of Severe Malnutrition Z score $SD \leq 3$ in the Cohort Subjects at Different Ages for Stunting, Underweight, and Wasting   134

3.3.3    Distribution for WHO Head Circumference at Different Age for Z Score $< -2$ in Cohort Subjects   135

3.3.4    Distribution for WHO MUAC for Age Z Score $< -2$ and $MUAC < 11.5$ in Different Age Groups of Cohort Subjects (UMAC Measurement is Available Only After 1.8 Years of Age)   136

6.1.1   Summary of Descriptive Variables for the Three Generations
        Among Age Group 4–12 Years of the NDBC                        202
6.1.2   Summary of Descriptive Variables for the Three Generations
        Among Age Group > 12 years of the NDBC                        203

7.1.1   Attrition in Various Phases of the NDBC Study                  214

# List of Figures

1.1.1  Founders of the NDBC                                          10
1.1.2  From Left to Right: Dr S. K. Bhargava, Dr S. Ghosh,
       Dr V. Hooja, and Dr S. K. Sanyal. Members of Paediatric
       Department                                                   17
1.1.3  Schedules Used for Primary Data Collection                   20
1.2.1  Registering the Cohort                                       25
1.3.1  Distribution of Families According to Number of Rooms
       in Different Areas                                           33
1.3.2  Depicting Linear Relationship Between Numbers of
       Foetal Loss/Child Death by Mean Number of Pregnancies        40
1.3.3  Distribution by Age and Family Planning Status               42
1.3.4  Family Planning Practices and Number of Pregnancies          44
1.3.5  Showing a Direct Increase in Non-users of Contraceptives
       with Increase in Child Mortality Experience                  45

2.2.1  Logo of the NDBC                                             54
2.2.2  Comparison of Distribution of Births at Different
       Gestation in NDBC and the USA                               55
2.2.3  Factors Influencing Gestation                               59
2.2.4  Percentile Intrauterine Growth Curve for Weight of the
       Cohort Subjects                                             64
2.2.5  Percentile Intrauterine Growth Curve for Length of the
       Cohort Subjects                                             64
2.2.6  Percentile Intrauterine Growth Curve for Head
       Circumference of the Cohort Subjects                        65
2.2.7  Comparison of Foetal Growth Curves for Birth Weight
       and Gestational Age of NDBC, Safdarjung Hospital, and
       INTERGROWTH-21                                              66
2.3.1  Distribution in Different Birth Weight Groups               70
2.3.2  Distribution by Birth Weight and Gestational Age            71

2.3.3   Neonatal Mortality Rate Per 1,000 Births in Different
Birth Weight Groups                                           74
2.3.4   Neonatal Mortality Rate Per 1,000 Births in Different
Birth Weight Groups by Gestation                             75
2.3.5   Birth Weight and Body Growth in Weight from Birth to
20 Years in Boys                                             79
2.3.6   Birth Weight and Body Growth in Weight from Birth to
20 Years in Girls                                            80
2.3.7   Birth Weight and Height from Birth to 20 Years in Boys   81
2.3.8   Small for Gestation and Body Growth in Body Weight
from Birth to 20 Years                                       82

3.1.1   Comparison of NDBC and IAP Percentile Curves in
Weight for Boys from 0 to 18 Years                          110
3.1.2   Comparison of NDBC and IAP Percentile Curves in
Weight for Girls from 0 to 18 Years                         111
3.1.3   Comparison of NDBC and IAP Percentile Curves in
Height for Boys from 0 to 18 Years                          112
3.1.4   Comparison of NDBC and IAP Percentile Curves in
Height for Girls from 0 to 18 Years                         113
3.1.5   Growth in Head Circumference of NDBC from Birth to
20 Years                                                    114
3.1.6   Percentile Growth in Head Circumference of NDBC
from Birth to 20 Years                                      115
3.1.7   Incremental Growth in Weight of NDBC from Birth to
20 Years                                                    118
3.1.8   Incremental Growths in Height of NDBC from Birth to
20 Years                                                    119
3.2.1   CD Scores in School Going and Not School Going
Children at 6 Years                                         128
3.3.1   Prevalence of Stunting, Underweight, and Wasting at
Different Age in Cohort Subjects                            135

4.1.1   The NDBC Research Group                                 139
4.2.1   The Adult Phase Research Group                          143
4.3.1   The Four Generations of the NDBC                        149
4.3.2   Cohorts in Different Phases of Study 1969–2015          151
4.3.3   Pre-field Clinic, Clinic, and Post-clinic Activities    153
4.3.4   Schedules/Pro Formas Used in the Adult Phase VI–VIII
Studies                                                     154

| 4.4.1 | Distribution for Water and Sanitation Facilities for F1 Cohort in Adult Phase | 157 |
| 4.4.2 | Education Pattern in F1 Cohort in Adult Phase | 158 |
| 4.4.3 | Occupation Patterns of F1 Cohorts in Adult Phase | 159 |
| 5.1.1 | Longitudinal BMI Trajectory in Diabetes | 167 |
| 5.1.2 | Longitudinal BMI Trajectories Till Adulthood in Subjects with High Blood Pressure, Low Systolic Blood Pressure, and Low Diastolic Blood Pressure | 168 |
| 5.1.3 | Longitudinal BMI Trajectories Till Adulthood in Subjects with High and Low Waist Hip Ratios (High Waist Hip Ratio) | 169 |
| 5.1.4 | Longitudinal BMI Trajectories Till Adulthood in Subjects with High and Low Serum Triglycerides | 169 |
| 6.0.1 | The Four Generations of the NDBC | 192 |
| 6.1.1 | Intergenerational Changes in Anthropometry | 194 |
| 6.1.2 | Birth Weight and LBW Intergenerational Change | 196 |
| 6.1.3 | Prevalence of Wasting in F1 and F2 Generation | 197 |
| 6.1.4 | Prevalence of Stunting in F1 and F2 Generations | 197 |
| 6.1.5 | Prevalence of Underweight in F1 and F2 Generations | 198 |
| 6.1.6 | Scatter Graph of BMI Change in F1 and F2 Generations | 200 |
| 6.2.1 | Cardiovascular Risk Factors in F2 Adolescences | 206 |

# List of Abbreviations

| | |
|---|---|
| aBMD | Areal Bone Mineral Density |
| AGA | Appropriate for Gestation Age |
| APOA5 | re-sequencing the Apolipoprotein A5 |
| BMAD | Bone Mineral Apparent Density |
| BCG | Bacille Calmette Guerin |
| BMC | Bone Mineral Content |
| BMI | Body Mass Index |
| BT20 | Birth to Twenty Study |
| CAD | Coronary Artery Disease |
| CBCL | Child Behaviour Check List |
| CBSE | Central Board of Secondary Education |
| CD | Cognitive Development |
| CDC | Centers for Disease Control and Prevention |
| CGAS | Children Global Assessment Scale |
| CGHS | Central Government Health Scheme |
| CHD | Coronary Heart Disease |
| CIE | Central Institute of Education |
| CIMT | Carotid Intima Media Thickness |
| COHORTS | Consortium of Health Research in Transitioning Societies |
| CT | Computed Tomography |
| CVS | Cardiovascular System |
| DEXA | Dual X-ray Absorptiometry |
| DPT | Diphtheria, Pertussis, and Tetanus |
| ECG | Electrocardiogram |
| ECHO | Echocardiography |
| GAD | Generalized Anxiety Disorder |
| GCC | Grand Challenges Canada |
| HDL | High-Density Lipoprotein |
| hsCRP | high-sensitivity C-Reactive Protein |

| | |
|---|---|
| IA-2 | Islet Antigen 2 |
| IAP | Indian Academy of Paediatrics |
| ICDS | Integrated Child Development Services |
| ICMR | Indian Council of Medical Research |
| IGT | Impaired Glucose Tolerance |
| INCAP | Institute of Nutrition of Central America and Panama |
| IQ | Intelligence Quotient |
| IUGR | Intrauterine Growth Retardation |
| LBW | Low Birth Weight |
| LDL | Low-Density Lipoprotein |
| LGA | Large for Gestation Age |
| LHV | Lady Health Visitors |
| LMP | Last Menstrual Period |
| MGRS | Multi-Country Growth Reference Study |
| MGRS | Multicentre Growth Reference Study |
| MRC | Medical Research Council |
| NCERT | National Council of Educational Research and Training |
| NCHS | National Centre for Health Statistics |
| NDBC | New Delhi Birth Cohort |
| NIDDM | Noninsulin-Dependent Diabetes Mellitus |
| OPD | OutPatient Department |
| PAI-1 | Plasminogen Activator Inhibitor-I |
| PHN | Public Health Nurse |
| PL 480 | Public Law 480 |
| PPARγ | Peroxisome Proliferator-Activated Receptor Gamma |
| SD | Standard Deviation |
| SGA | Small for Gestation Age |
| SNEHA | Society for Nutrition Education and Health Action |
| UK | United Kingdom |
| UMAC | Upper Mid-arm Circumference |
| USA | United States of America |
| UNICEF | United Nations Children's Fund |
| USAID | United States Agency for International Development |
| WHO | World Health Organization |

# Foreword

Of all human relationships, the bond between mother and child is the most precious—sanctified in religion, celebrated in literature, glorified in art, and affirmed by science as the essential key to the survival and sustenance of the human race. The health of mothers and children features prominently in both the Millennium Development Goals of 2000 and the Sustainable Development Goals of 2015. Concerns about their health and commitments for action are not only related to prevention of avertable deaths but also to the promotion of good health and nutrition. It is now well recognized that the nutritional states of a pregnant woman, the baby in her womb, and the growing infant not only portray strong intergenerational links among themselves but also profile the strong connectivity that courses across lives, from the preconception nutrition and growth of the adolescent girl to the adulthood of her offspring. Indeed, there is now growing evidence that epigenetic changes resulting from intrauterine or early childhood malnutrition could exert their health effects even in the progeny of the progeny. Understanding these links, and acting to promote adequate and appropriate nutrition at each stage, is pivotal to the global health and development agenda.

Much of this knowledge has been generated in the past few decades through cohort studies that have followed women and their children through pregnancy, birth and, later, life. One of the early birth cohort studies was initiated in India, in New Delhi, in 1969. It was originally intended to study the problem of low birth weight (LBW) and its sequelae. It was a remarkable testament to the scientific vision and vigour of paediatricians from the Safdarjung Hospital. Later, research by David Barker and other scientists revealed that poor nutrition in the womb and early childhood, which manifest as LBW and size as well as sub-optimal growth in infancy, were linked to increased risk of diabetes and cardiovascular diabetes in adult life—often with an early onset of chronic disease. The New Delhi Birth Cohort (NDBC) was then reassembled and followed through to the current phase where it includes four generations. Through meticulous trans-disciplinary research that links scientists from several institutions across the world, the NDBC has unravelled many links and elucidated key mechanisms underlying the developmental origins of adult disease, especially throwing light on how 'rebound adiposity' and relative weight gain in later years of childhood can propel an LBW baby into the high-risk zone of cardiometabolic diseases in adulthood.

Dr Santosh Bhargava, the lead scientist associated with this study since its inception, describes the fascinating story of how this cohort was assembled and followed over nearly half a century. He narrates the key findings that emerged at each stage of the study and cites the highly impactful scientific publications that flowed from them into leading medical journals across the world. This, and similar research from other parts of the world, has led to a major global scientific movement around Developmental Origins of Health and Disease (DOHAD). This movement is dedicated to the advancement of knowledge on the effects of maternal and child nutrition across the life course, as a human embryo journeys from a woman's womb to the wide world to experience various stages of growth and further development. Based on this growing body of scientific knowledge, DOHAD also provides valuable recommendations for public health action.

India needs to pay heed to such research and resolutely implement public health measures to promote women's nutrition—before, during, and after pregnancy—and ensure protective nutrition for children at all stages of their growth. This is especially important as India still has unconscionably high levels of underweight or stunted children, while experiencing the rapidly escalating burdens of diabetes and cardiovascular disease. As the evidence presented by this book shows, these are interrelated, with malnutrition in early life casting a long and dark shadow over health in later life. We need to act at all critical intervention points to interrupt this intergenerational carryover of nutritional disadvantage and avert the many health hazards of damaged child development.

Dr Bhargava brings to this book the scientific objectivity of a researcher, the caring sensitivity of a paediatrician and the conviction of a writer who wishes to use his pen to stir societal conscience. It makes a compelling reading for anyone interested in the health and well-being of India's children.

**K. Srinath Reddy**
President, Public Health Foundation of India

# Preface

There is an ancient Sanskrit proverb—*Bhavti Bhavtu*—which means that if something has to happen it will happen. The establishment of the NDBC had to happen and it happened. Also, if one is a believer of coincidences, then the story of 'the NDBC' from its foundation in 1969 to its successful continuation in its 48th year is a good example. Its inception was by the coincidence of the publication of two similar articles on birth weight and gestational age in the same journal by Dr Yerushalmy from the USA and Dr Shanti Ghosh from India. Both of them were deeply interested in birth weight, gestation, and outcome of births. It seemed incidental to have the initial PL 480 funds for Indo–US research projects to start the cohort as also the subsequent repeated extensions after an initial 4-year grant was completed. This enabled the evaluation of varying objectives from birth to adulthood by funding primarily from the National Centre for Health and Statistics, USA, and the Indian Council of Medical Research, India.

The revival of the cohort in 1995 too was by coincidence. Dr Anand Pandit from Pune had casually mentioned the NDBC to Professor David Barker, which led to a meeting between him and Professor Bhargava, one of the founders of the NDBC (writer) in Delhi at the 8th Asian Congress of Paediatrics. Their mutual interest in the problem and determination to revive the cohort during adulthood to test the Barker's hypothesis of foetal origin of adult diseases thus evolved from a chance mention.

The biggest coincidence was the finding and recovery of the original 29 magnetic tapes containing the data records of the first 20 years of research, which were believed to have been lost after intense search. These were found in a store under a table without any label or information as to what these tapes stored. It was also sheer luck that the computer scientist Dr Dey Biswas happened to bring his daughter for medical consultation to Dr Bhargava who casually asked for his help in the analysis of these data tapes. It was also a stroke of luck that the first tape, number

28, which was opened by Dr Dey Biswas, contained the contact details of the cohort. Breaking the data codes of these magnetic tapes needed a monumental effort, expertise and patience. Further research emanated from different grants from planned or accidental meetings with interested collaborators and investigators.

The NDBC was established to investigate the problem of LBW in India. It not only investigated the initial objectives but also completed a unique life-course study on LBW. Over time, the objectives were expanded to study body growth from birth to 20 years, at age specific periods, and construct reference growth curves from birth, to childhood, to adolescence and adulthood.

The nature of data collection, records, and analysis stimulated further research into body growth, body composition, and its influence on development of adult diseases such as diabetes, hypertension, coronary and carotid artery diseases, and metabolic syndrome. Barker's hypothesis of foetal origin of adult diseases, now known as the developmental origin of adult diseases, was also tested.

The body growth data led to a further collaboration with four similar cohorts, Pelotas from Brazil, the Institute of Nutrition of Central America and Panama (INCAP) from Guatemala, Cebu from Philippines, and the Birth to Twenty Study (BT20) from South Africa. This collaboration of five cohorts from low- and middle-income countries was given the acronym COHORTS (Consortium of Health Research in Transitioning Societies). The collaboration examined the data for the influence of birth weight and the body growth from early and middle childhood to adolescence and adulthood on several outcomes including impaired glucose tolerance, diabetes, metabolic syndrome, and human capital development.

This COHORTS group established the influence of maternal nutrition, foetal growth, and growth in the first two years to be optimal for human capital development (adult stature, schooling outcome, income generation, and the effect on the birth weight of the next offspring of women). This contributed to the coining of the term the 'first 1,000 days'. The collaborative research further showed the effect of rapid growth and rapid gain in body mass index (BMI) after four years of age leading to adiposity or fatness. The research also established the need to monitor growth meticulously, interpret it, and intervene, as it is possible to track adult diseases such as diabetes, metabolic syndrome, hypertension, overweight and obesity, and others by tracking them from as early as birth, infancy, and through childhood.

During its journey, the NDBC has expanded from a one-generation cohort to a four-generation one—F0 are the parents of the cohort, F1 are the cohorts, F2 are the children of the cohorts, and F3 are the grandchildren of cohorts. This allowed an insight into intergeneration and trans-generational changes in anthropometry, nutrition, cardiometabolic risk factors and specific diseases in the F2 generation or the children of cohorts.

Ascribing everything to luck, chance, and coincidence would belittle the vast contributions of the cohort subjects and their families, the NDBC collaborators from many countries and institutions, the research team, the institution heads and administrators, and many others. It was through their conjoint efforts, understanding and commitment that the NDBC is continuing and contributing to highly relevant research at the national and global levels.

This book is intended to chronicle, in brief, the experiences in setting up the NDBC and its continuation into the fifth decade of existence and also document the salient research findings, particularly those of importance for national policy and practice. This could prove to be a valuable resource for researchers planning to establish new cohorts, paediatricians, obstetricians, adult physicians, cardiologists, endocrinologists, demographers, social scientists, public health administrators, economists, policy-makers, and other stakeholders in national health issues.

# Acknowledgements

It is with fond remembrance and profound and heartfelt gratitude that I wish to acknowledge the far-sighted vision and contribution made by my mentor the late Professor Dr Shanti Ghosh, the founder of the NDBC. But for her understandings of the country's child health issues, her recognition of prematurity, and LBW as a major public health problem and her sustained research in it, the NDBC would never have been founded.

To late Dr I. M. Moriyama, the other co-founder of the cohort, I owe an immeasurable debt for being a philosopher, guide, and a friend, who with his gentle nature, deep insight into research, and eye for detail taught me the relevance of being patient, consistent, and focused.

I have been very fortunate to work and be associated with several leading researchers of national and international eminence by their collaboration and active participation in various projects of the NDBC. They are too numerous, and it is an impossible task to acknowledge everyone's contribution and thank each one of them individually. But I wish to put on record my sincere thanks to all of them for their help, involvement, and support in the journey of the NDBC.

I am extremely grateful to late Professor David Barker who initiated us into investigation of the Barker's hypothesis of 'foetal origin of adult diseases' in the NDBC subjects. This further resulted in a very successful and productive collaboration with Professor Caroline Fall and Professor Clive Osmond, which led to several studies on determining the influence of birth weight and childhood growth on cardiometabolic disorders. I am extremely thankful to them for their continued support and association during the last two decades.

It seemed providential to meet Professor C. Victora, Professor L. Richter, Professor Reynolds Martorell, and Professor L. Adair leading similar cohorts from low middle-income countries and to form the 'COHORTS' group, which contributed to numerous studies on maternal and child health and nutrition and their influence on adult health, disease, and human capital. I feel honoured to have been a part of the group and feel grateful to them for their continued support and collaboration.

Professor K.S. Reddy's perceptive foreword captures the spirit of the book and his association with the NDBC has been a guiding force from the adult phase of the studies. I was also fortunate to work with Professor H. P. S. Sachdev, Professor S. Ramji, Professor D. Prabhakaran, Professor N. Tandon, Professor R. Lakshmy, Dr S. K. Dey Biswas, Professor A. Khalil, Professor Rajesh Sagar, Dr Poornima Prabhakaran, and Dr T. Gera and get their active support, participation, and help in the successful completion of various projects of the NDBC. I will always remain very thankful to all of them.

The NDBC is a unique success story of a birth cohort running since the past five decades and is still ongoing. This is largely because it has been blessed with a team of dedicated and committed researchers who have always regarded the NDBC as their own project and gave it their best in terms of time, energy, loyalty, and commitment. In the beginning, it was led by Dr Vijay Hooja, who had set the standards of fieldwork by the motto 'Cohort first and Cohort last.' Ms Rajeshwari Verma continued the tradition and was responsible in retracing the cohorts in the adult phase and re-establishing the NDBC. Mr Bhaskar Singh holds the mantle now, and with him are many other field staff and other colleagues who have been largely responsible for successfully continuing it in last 20 years. I express my sincere thanks to all of them.

A birth cohort of NDBC's nature is bound to be a repository and wealth of research documents, data, and information, and it is due to the foresight of the data managers and experts that the NDBC continues to be relevant for contemporary research and analysis. I owe it all to Dr A. D. Taskar, Dr Shantha Madhavan, Mr Ramanujam and Ms Rita Tulsany who laid the foundation of the data repository in the founding years and thereafter to the dedication and hard work of Mr Vinod Kapani who managed the huge data, and stored, analysed, and compiled it as documents and reports. I am grateful to all of them, especially to Mr Kapani for his huge support and advice and for access and use of his report. I sincerely thank my former colleagues, late Dr S. C. Khandpur, late Dr Man Mohan and Dr S. S. Uppal, who have been investigators in the childhood phase and for their contribution to the project and its completion.

I am thankful to Dr S. K. Dey Biswas who single-handedly retrieved the original data from the magnetic tapes which had their data directory lost. Professor H. P. S. Sachdev, ably supported by Ms Sikha Sinha, has been the custodian of the NDBC data repository. He has steered the complex data analysis with his clarity of thoughts and expertise, which has largely laid the foundation for the NDBC publications.

The journey of the NDBC with the perpetual uncertainty of research funds, and my own struggles of life in trying to be successful in many of my other preoccupations and commitments, could not have been completed but for the support, drive, and assurance which I unfailingly received from my colleagues, friends, and family. Dr S. K. Sanyal and Dr H. M. K. Saxena motivated me to encompass research with my clinical responsibilities in my formative years. Professor H. P. S. Sachdev and Professor S. Ramji always gave me invaluable advice and support at the NDBC with its numerous research projects in which we were a part of collaborations. I deeply appreciate this and remain particularly grateful to Professor Sachdev for being my support while writing this book, reviewing the manuscript and for his critical incisive comments. I am grateful to Mr Bhaskar Singh for his help in preparing the manuscript of this book, in the literature search and the selection of photographs, figures, and drawings. I am very thankful to Ms Rita Joseph who had to bear the major burden from the preparatory stage—typing drafts, finding files, and keeping track of the enormous paper work and notes involved while writing this book.

I am extremely grateful to Ms Sunanda Ghosh, who encouraged me to write this book and constantly helped with her constructive and valuable advice.

I am very thankful to the Seth Sunder Lal Jain Charitable Eye Hospital Society and Sunder Lal Jain Hospital for providing the NDBC its office, and to Mr V. K. Jain for administrative support and constant guidance and help.

I am grateful to late Professor J. Yerushalmy and the scientific section of the US embassy in establishing and then sustaining the project by grants from the US National Center for Health Statistics, USA, and the PL 480 funds, India, and to The Indian Council of Medical Research, particularly its Director Generals Dr C. Gopalan and Dr V. Ramalingaswamy, for providing timely support by bridging grants for completion of the childhood phase of the project. I thank the British Heart Foundation; Wessex Medical Trust; Southampton General Hospital, Southampton; Medical Research Council, Southampton; Wellcome Trust, UK; Department of Biotechnology and the Department of Science & Technology, Government of India, India; Bill & Melinda Gates Foundation; Emory and Stanford University, USA; and the Institute of Developmental Sciences, New Zealand for research grants and support.

It would have been impossible for me to write the book without the support of my family who suffered due to my commitment and preoccupation with the NDBC from its foundation days. My wife Manorama has been my inspiration and pillar of strength; my children Sumit and Shibani the impetus who always said 'go for it'; Anna, my daughter-in-law, and Hiren, my-son-in-law, who as readers offered their inputs on the manuscript. Every single word of encouragement and suggestion helped me to sustain my self-belief in writing and completing the story of the NDBC.

I am thankful to SAGE Publications for agreeing to publish this book and to its team for their constant guidance and help.

# Introduction

After centuries of oppression and deprivation, India is currently undergoing a transition of an economic resurgence and a nutritional shift from undernutrition to overnutrition. While in the earlier period it had a large burden of childhood morbidity and mortality caused by underweight, it is now facing the problems and consequences of overweight and obesity from children to adults. India has a very high prevalence of low birth weight (LBW). The country has not been able to plan and develop an effective strategy to deal with this problem due to lack of evidence from prospective, large-community-based studies. It is in this context the birth cohort study on which this book is based was planned and initiated. Cohort studies were uncommon in those days as these were considered difficult to sustain, were expansive and needed huge effort. However, considering the nature of the widely prevalent problem of low birth in the country and the paucity of reliable epidemiologic data, it was decided to undertake the project. It proved a very valuable and farsighted decision. As the study evolved, it was able to investigate the development of chronic adult cardiometabolic diseases from childhood to adulthood. India is considered the world capital of diabetes with its rapidly increasing prevalence. It is also expected to increase several fold along with cardiovascular diseases to become a leading cause of adult deaths.

The narrative of this book travels across five decades capturing the transiting changes in socio-economic fabric, economic prosperity, and nutritional abundance. It attempts to describe in an urban cohort the actual prevalence, emergence of adult diseases, and positive changes which are now occurring trans-generationally. It offers suggestions for tracking, prevention, and intervention from early childhood for the threatening adult cardiometabolic disorders.

The cohort was established in 1969. It was to determine the extent of the burning public health problem of low birth, what contributed to its causation and its outcome in terms of immediate and late survival and sequelae. The need arose as almost 1/3–1/2 of the babies were being born with a birth weight less than 2.5 kg. These were not a homogenous group but comprised premature and/or intrauterine-growth-retarded infants. A large number of these infants died, contributing to very high infant and childhood mortality. It was not even known as to what happened to those who survived and whether they were afflicted with challenging physical or mental problems in later life.

The study is based on a large urban community cohort and describes the demographic features for those times, which provide an insight into the social practices, environmental conditions, and family life and records changes occurring over several decades. This was also the time when the country was becoming aware of the problem of population explosion and the national government was aggressively advocating adoption of family planning practices. The study offers an insight into the fertility pattern and family planning practices, and highlights the effect of pregnancy loss and child mortality on adoption of family welfare programme by the couples.

This study is based on a large community cohort and allows follow-up and comparison of both normal and LBW children. This offered an opportunity to record their outcome in normal course of their lives for survival, illness, and well-being through infancy to adulthood. A wealth of information became available on health care practices in pregnancy and childbirth care, utilization of health care facilities, and implementation of government programmes and general health care. It documents the prevailing status of maternal and child health, immunization practices, and their acceptance by the community. The study provides a large sample of LBW children and gives an account of the factors and causes contributing to it, their mortality and morbidity pattern, and consequences of being born small over a life course. It accorded a chance to study undernutrition in detail and observe the magnitude of the problem and its effects through childhood and in later life. It allowed testing the cognitive development (CD) abilities in children, and the influence of birth weight and other factors affecting these in natural and home surroundings. One of the highlights of the book is the description of growth pattern of children from birth through different periods of childhood and adolescence until attainment of adulthood. It provides growth charts for normal children, body composition at different age periods, and age-independent indices for assessment of growth. One of the most important gains has been to investigate and compare the health outcomes of normal and low birth children over five decades.

In 1986, a most interesting study was published by Barker and colleagues who reported an association between infant mortality, childhood nutrition, and ischaemic heart disease, and found it more commonly in the poorest areas of England. In seminal publications, they reported the association of LBW with coronary artery disease and propounded the Barker's hypothesis of 'foetal origin of adult disease'. He suggested that the adverse influences, especially during intrauterine period, resulted in permanent changes in body physiology and metabolism, which lead to chronic cardiovascular and metabolic diseases in adult lives.

During this period, India has been going through an economic, epidemiological, and nutrition change. The study initiated in 1969 had been through the transiting changes as it covers a period of over three decades and is ongoing. The birth cohorts had prospectively and meticulously collected data from the urban community from preconception to conception, childbirth, and at age-specific periods for body growth and body composition. In 1998, we got an opportunity to test Barker's hypothesis now known as developmental origin of health and adult disease through a collaborative study with Professor Barker and Professor Fall in the subjects of the New Delhi Birth Cohort (NDBC). We determined the association of birth weight and body growth with the development of diabetes, hypertension, and other metabolic disorders in young adult between 26 and 29 years of age and again later during their follow-up till the current age. The findings were surprising, with high prevalence of these diseases beginning at a young age. The major finding was the susceptibility of thin children who became overweight or fat to these disorders. The study highlighted the possibility of identifying these children by their rapid increase in body mass index (BMI) on standard growth charts.

The influence of birth weight, body growth, and body composition have now become major areas of interest and concern for health care providers and policy planners. These have been extensively studied, analysed and reviewed in this book and form one of the major high points of this monograph. A low or high birth weight and rapid or slow growth at different periods of childhood can all be detrimental to health in adulthood. These in addition to body composition measurements at different periods have shown a relationship to adult disease like obesity and metabolic syndrome. One of the major findings has been documenting the positive gains of optimal growth during intrauterine period and the first two years of life—coined as 'The first 1,000 days'—to be critical for human development. The detrimental effect of rapid growth from preschool years through childhood period and its correlation with adult disease points to the importance of growth monitoring from conception to adulthood as an important, practical and simple tool to anticipate and prevent adult diseases.

In five decades of its journey, the consortium of health research in transitioning societies (cohort) from a single generation study has become a family cohort with four generations. It offers an opportunity to record the intergenerational changes in environment, socio-economic condition, body growth, and nutrition. It shows the gain of the economic prosperity through an increase in wealth index, which was associated with decrease in LBW and increase in body weight, height, and BMI. It records a generational change in nutritional status in children under five. But the alarming aspect which is of great concern is an increase in early and significant occurrence of adult diseases such as obesity and hypertension in young adolescence children. It records trans-generation deterioration in the metabolic profile across three generations of the cohorts.

In essence, the book depicts the Indian story of a birth cohort in association with similar cohorts in other low- and middle-income countries, and the impact of birth weight and childhood growth on adult health and human capital. It suggests growth monitoring as a simple tool to anticipate and prevent the onslaught of chronic adult disease affecting the quality of human life.

# PART 1

# Background of the Study

# 1

# Genesis

## Introduction

Birth weight and the growth of children from birth to adulthood has always remained an area of concern for parents, policy-makers, health providers, and researchers. When a child is born, amongst the first few questions that the parents and families ask is about the birth weight and then as the child grows about its being small or big. The perennial question asked is about the consequences, if any, of impaired growth and small or tall stature. The story of the NDBC over a life course is also about these two prime concerns—the size at birth and the body growth and its immediate or late consequences in life.

All over the world, especially in the developing countries like India, public health authorities are becoming aware of the health problems due to rapid nutrition transition and lifestyle changes and their adverse consequences in adult lives. The importance of birth weight for immediate outcome has always been known for centuries, but as survival of premature and LBW infants improved, its sequelae in childhood and adolescence became an area of intense interest and research in the latter half of the last century. It was established that the smaller the size of the baby, the greater the risk to life and poor health [1–15]. But the implication of a small size or LBW with rapid body growth in childhood and its association with adult diseases has only been recognised in the last 2–3 decades [16–20].

In the last century, the debate revolved around the definition and criteria for cut-off for birth weight, and for identifying LBW for special care and its accompanying risk and care. But in recent years, the rapidly changing socio-environment, nutrition, economic gains and education, and vastly improved living conditions with sedentary life have been identified as the major contributing factors for middle and old age morbidities and mortality due to adult metabolic and cardiovascular diseases.

In India and the developing world, Dr Shanti Ghosh spearheaded the debate on defining LBW criterion and definition in the 1950s and the 1960s [21]. She and others pointed out that if the World Health Organization (WHO) definition of all infants with birth weight of less than 2,500 g for LBW weight is accepted, then 30–50% of newborn infants will be premature or termed LBW. Thus, every other newborn will be categorized for the need of special care or admission to special care nurseries and baby care units. This would be in sharp contrast to the developed world where only about 10% of newborns with birth weight less than 2,500 g are either premature or LBW. She showed from her extensive in-depth research from New Delhi, India, that mortality and morbidities such as delayed cry (asphyxia), breast and other methods of feeding difficulties, and infections sharply declined at birth weight of 4 lb (Pounds) or 2 kg (kilogram) and above. She argued that most of the newborn infants between 4 lb and 5 and a 1/2 lb or 2,000–2,500 g did not need special care and could be looked after under supervised care by the mother. She therefore suggested that for India and the developing world, a cut-off point of 4 lb or 2,000 g or less would be a more appropriate, practical, and reasonable criterion for defining LBW. If this definition was applied, then only about 10% of newborns would need a special care nursery admission, which was comparable to developed western countries LBW prevalence (< 2,500 g) and need of special care nurseries. Similar concerns and views were also expressed by paediatricians from several South East Asian countries such as by de Silva from Sri Lanka [21].

Dr Shanti Ghosh continued her work on birth weight and gestation to strengthen her argument and belief that the outcome of Indian infants, which are born LBW and/or premature, need Indian standards and not international as recommended by WHO and developed counties from the West. In an interesting coincidence, she published her paper 'Comparisons of Gestational Age and Weight as Standards of Prematurity' in the *Journal of Paediatrics* [22]. Similar papers though from a vastly different developed country like the USA by Yerushalmy entitled 'The Classification of Newborn Infants by Birth Weight and Gestational Age' in the *Journal of Paediatrics* [23] and Battaglia and

Lubchanco entitled 'A Practical Classification of Newborn Infants by Weight and Gestational Age' also appeared in the same issue of the *Journal of Paediatrics* [24]. These papers presented evidence from their respective countries on birth weight and gestation distribution and their importance and relevance in classifying mortality and morbidity patterns.

Soon after the publication of these articles, an interesting development happened. Dr Dorothy Cooke, Chief, International Research Branch Office of the International Statistical Programmes of the Department of Health, Education and Welfare, Washington DC, USA, wrote to Dr Shanti Ghosh, Head, Department of Paediatrics, Safdarjung Hospital, on 14 August 1967 indicating Dr Jacob Yerushalmy's, Professor of Biostatistics, University of California, interest in a collaborative study. Dr Cooke visited India and met Dr Ghosh on 17 August 1967 in Delhi. It was decided by them to have further discussions with Dr Yerushalmy on the feasibility of a joint project on the problem of LBW in India. After several meetings between Dr Yerushalmy, Dr Ghosh, Dr A. D. Taskar, Head, Division of Biostatistics, Indian Council of Medical Research (ICMR), Dr Santosh K. Bhargava, Paediatrician, Safdarjung Hospital (author), and others, it was decided to formally apply for a research grant under the Public Law 480 (PL 480) scheme of the Governments of India and the United States of America (USA).

A draft proposal was then prepared by Dr Ghosh and submitted to the ICMR for onward transmission to Dr J. Yerushalmy for further consideration in the USA. The initial objectives included standards of prematurity and LBW survival and their growth, development, and congenital malformations.

The project was approved in principle, and further discussions and meetings were then held between investigators from the USA and India, the ICMR, and officials of the American embassy in India for a final proposal.

At this time, a similar project was being developed by Dr J. Yerushalmy and Dr K. S. Sunder Rao, Head, Department of Biochemistry, Christian Medical College, Vellore. It was decided to have two independent project officers for the two projects from the USA and from India. Dr J. Yerushalmy became the projector officer for the Vellore project with Dr K. S. Sunder Rao as the principal investigator.

Dr I. M. Moriyama, Statistician, National Centre for Health and Statistics, USA, became the project officer for the New Delhi project with Dr Shanti Ghosh as principal investigator and Dr Santosh K. Bhargava

**Figure 1.1.1:**
*Founders of the NDBC*

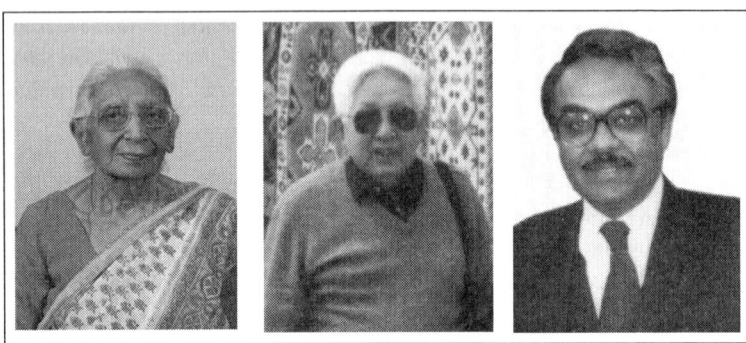

|  Dr Shanti Ghosh | Dr I. M. Moriyama | Dr Santosh K. Bhargava |

*Source:* Author.

as co-investigator for the project entitled 'Longitudinal Study of the Survival and Outcome of a Birth Cohort' with a grant from Research Project 01-658-2, funded by the National Centre for Health Statistics, USA (NCHS), and funded the NDBC (Figure 1.1.1).

## Planning of the Study

The project had been an outcome of the interest of Dr Ghosh, Dr Bhargava, and Dr Yerushalmy in LBW with special focus on birth weight, gestation, and foetal growth retardation. The initial objectives, therefore, focussed on these aspects, and the project was developed largely on the problem of LBW in the Indian context.

## Selection of Population

The selection of population for investigation had to be discussed in-depth as no similar study was ever done before in India or a similar low-income, developing country. It was finally decided that it had to be a prospective cohort-based study. Several options for cohort selection were then considered.

The first consideration was to take the index cases from the Safdarjung Hospital, New Delhi. This is a large government general hospital situated in South Delhi. It had about 7,000–8,000 deliveries every year. The mothers and their babies were to be followed from birth and then in the subsequent pregnancy. The birth of the next infant in these enrolled women would then provide the cohort for the study. This infant was to be followed prospectively as a birth cohort. As Safdarjung Hospital catered to a large area in and around Delhi, only 4,000 or so mothers residing in a well-defined area near the hospital were to be included for the study. While the use of hospital index cases would have provided important advantages for a cohort study with complete obstetrical and paediatric data, several limitations were also recognized. The main objections were unreliable gestational age data, absence of *primigravida* pregnancies, retrospective and biased nature of information, and inclusion of about 10% or more of complicated pregnancies which usually deliver at the hospital. The cohort may also not be representative of all the socio-economic groups as a vast majority of women from higher income groups preferred to go to private hospitals and nursing homes for delivery rather than come to a government hospital. It would also have been difficult to foresee the size of the second cohort of babies which was to form the main subjects of the study. It was therefore decided to explore the possibility of a prospective cohort study in a community rather than in a hospital.

We then considered the central government employee's population, as Delhi is the seat of the Central Government of India, which has a large population of these employees. They are covered by a prepaid health scheme known as the Central Government Health Scheme (CGHS) and are attached to a CGHS dispensary in their residential area. Each central government dispensary catered to a population of about 10,000 beneficiaries or so. Hence, it was estimated that beneficiaries allotted to 12 dispensaries would provide a population of 120,000, yielding about 20,755 women of childbearing age. These were expected to have about 8,100 newborn babies, calculated at the assumed birth rate of 40/1,000 prevalent at that time. However, when the preliminary survey was done, several unforeseen problems were encountered. It was found that the beneficiaries cards, kept at the dispensary, were not really the live cards. Several families had moved out of the area and the records were not updated. Of the 100 addresses noted from the cards, only 10 families could be traced. The attempts to get the much-needed information on numbers and addresses from the director general of CGHS also did not yield any results as their records were as outdated as those of the dispensaries.

Another method of tracing the beneficiaries was then tried at a few dispensaries situated within 3–4 km of Safdarjung Hospital. One public health nurse (PHN) was posted to each dispensary to note down the names of the heads of the households along with the complete addresses and details of the family members of those attending the dispensary. This was done with a view to obtain an accurate family history and census of the area. However, after carrying the survey for nearly a month, it was realized that this will not yield the desired results as the families that did not visit the dispensary, had better health, or went elsewhere for medical care would be left out of the study. Thus, it would result in a bias. This approach was therefore also rejected.

The next attempt was try to study the families living in government housing. Although the allotment of government accommodation would be a prerequisite and would result in bias as the government accommodation costs much less to hire (about one fourth or one fifth of the private hired housing), it would have the definite advantage of properly numbered houses and streets so that no household would be missed, ensuring better follow-up. However, we had disappointment in store here as well. The survey in two government colonies revealed that Laxmibai Nagar was housing mostly class III employees or the low-middle-class civil servants consisting mainly of clerical staff, and Kasturba Nagar was housing mostly class IV employees of the government working as sweepers, peons, watchmen etc. and their families. These populations would have been very selective and hence unsuitable.

Soon we encountered a very peculiar problem in Laxmibai Nagar. The population in the government colony belonged to an older age group (only 35% of women were below 35 years of age) as the government accommodation is allotted on the basis of seniority in service. Thus, the majority of couples already had the number of children they wanted. This would have resulted in low birth rate, causing problems in the reflection of vital statistics and the required number of cohort sample size.

In Kasturba Nagar, a different type of problem was encountered. In many houses, as many as 4 to 6 men were staying while their families were in the villages. Since the women folk did not stay in Delhi, no purpose would have been served by selecting this population. Moreover, during the preliminary survey, the field staff often found a woman in some houses who was supposed to be a cousin or a niece, and discretion in questioning seemed a sensible policy.

Other problems encountered in these colonies included the inability to obtain the names of the head of the household who was allotted the accommodation from the Ministry of Works and Housing and was subletting the house to non-central government employee. The truth about subletting was also not reported correctly as it was an offence and the breaking of government rules invited penalties and prosecution. So, the plan of studying the population in these government colonies had to be abandoned.

The selection of an industrial township called Faridabad which is 30 km from Safdarjung Hospital and where the refugees from the North West Frontier Province (part of Pakistan) were rehabilitated after partition of the Indian subcontinent was also considered. The distance from Safdarjung Hospital was a difficult problem and the township was situated in the adjoining state of Haryana. The permission of Haryana government would have delayed the initiation of the project considerably. The then Director General of Health Services, Government of India, also advised against it.

## Selection of Area

It was finally decided to locate the project in Lajpat Nagar (Part I, II, III, and IV) and add the adjacent colonies to it to have the target of 100,000 population. Reliable population data of this area was not available as the last census was eight years old. The estimates for population of Lajpat Nagar varied from 60,000 to 115,000. Even the Municipal Corporation of Delhi under whose jurisdiction this area is, was not sure about the population. Hence, it became imperative to conduct a fresh census of the area. This area consisted of the population which full filled the criterion for selection of the population. It was possible to obtain complete information on population characteristics including family profile, environment, social, and biological factors; women of reproductive age; urban population representative of all socio-economic strata; and it was close to Safdarjung Hospital.

## Pro Forma Development

While the selection of population was going on, an opportunity was taken to test the pro forma regarding their suitability and feasibility in two areas of the project. In Kasturba Nagar, several houses were contacted daily but only 4–5 households' pro forma could be filled as the head of the household was often away on work and the family was in the village. In Laxmibai Nagar, 10–12 families could be registered within a five-hour working schedule. The household, person, pregnant, and the non-pregnant women's pro forma as well as the pro forma pertaining to the baby were filled and tested. Repeat visits were made after two months in the case of both the pregnant and the non-pregnant women. In the light of the experience gained, the pro forma were suitably modified before finalizing them for study.

This testing exercise additionally gave an indication of the workload that each interviewer and PHN would be able to carry out. This helped in determining the number of interviewers and PHNs that would be needed for the project.

## Procuring Tools and Equipment for the Project

Procuring the right kind of tools and equipment for the project caused great concern and posed many problems. These were primarily due to non-availability of simple yet essential and appropriate kind of equipment such as infant weighing scales, infantometers for measuring length, and tapes for measuring different parts of the body such as head and chest circumference in the Indian market. Indian make instruments were not suitable for research purpose as these were not of standard quality and accuracy. The import of such equipment was not permitted by the national government because of severe foreign exchange constrains. Moreover, an undertaking was required to be given by the investigators of all PL-480 funded projects that no foreign exchange would be used or required. The most pressing problem was that of the infant weighing scales and infantometers to measure the length of the babies and record the weight. A wooden infantometer—a copy of the United Nations Children's Fund (UNICEF) model—was ordered as a sample but was found inaccurate and unsatisfactory.

Dr Indra Pal Singh, Professor of anthropology, Delhi University, came to our rescue and introduced us to Mr A. P. Jain, an anthropologist turned manufacturer of anthropometrics instruments. He devised an aluminium infantometer for us with 1 mm calibration and a stainless steel standiometer for measuring height. These were fairly sturdy instruments, able to withstand rough handling in the field. Aluminium and stainless steel was specially chosen for accuracy of measuring length and height since the expansion due to heat is negligible. Some improvements were made in the subsequent models. Procurement of weighing scales also posed a problem. Suitable lever types of scale were not available in the market and we failed to get them from agencies such as the ICMR, WHO, UNICEF, etc. An infant weighing scale of the Detecto kind was designed and manufactured locally by Mr Jain. These scales had the capacity to weigh only up to 10 kg but at least this enabled us to initiate the work. Later, three weighting scales were acquired through the courtesy of the United States Agency for International Development (USAID). Luckily, during 1971, Detecto-type scales with a capacity to weigh babies up to 16 kg became available in Delhi. However, the problem of weighing the older babies continued to pose a problem throughout. The steel measuring tapes (mollimex) for measuring the head and the chest circumference were easily available at first, but became scarce during the third and fourth year of the project.

The instruments were frequently checked against standard equipment for accuracy. In case a defect was noted, the instrument was discarded. The instruments were fabricated only once as the same became available in the later part of the study.

## Statistical and Data Management Tools and Equipment

Procuring data management tools and equipment was one of the most difficult tasks for the project and it resulted in several hurdles. It required the staff to do the hard work manually. To begin with, it was planned that the entire data would be punched and recorded for computer analysis. Hence, the pro forma and data collection methods for the staff were designed accordingly. But the project could not even procure a calculating machine as the same were not available in the Indian market. The project was bound by import restrictions and, hence, initially all the data was recorded manually and the calculations were done with adding machines or manually.

The project in its budget and planning had provided for the IBM automatic punching and verifying machine which arrived only in the middle of the second year. Dr Yerushalmy gifted a broken calculating machine which was repaired towards the end of the second year, which was a blessing. It resolved many day-to day-problems of calculations and helped in analysis and preparing reports.

## Locating the Project Staff and Administrative Office

Accommodation for the project office also posed a problem. It would not have been easy to rent accommodation in a suitable place near the hospital. Besides, it would have meant considerable extra expense for rent, electricity, water, maintenance, and some help for cleaning etc. which was not provided in the budget. The investigators would have required considerable time for traveling between the hospital and the project office. Transport would have been an additional problem. Dr P. P. Goel, medical superintendent of the Safdarjung Hospital, generously made some accommodation available in two locations. The field staff was located in a large corridor of the outpatient department (OPD) wing of the Department of Paediatrics and the administrative and secretarial office in a ward near the principal investigator, Dr Ghosh's department office. This was extremely convenient for supervision, administration, and monitoring of the project.

## Recruitment of Staff

This was begun in March 1969. The two senior research officers, one paediatrician and one statistician were selected on 10 February 1969. The project was fortunate in securing the services or Mrs Shantha Madhavan as senior statistician who joined the project in April 1969 on deputation from the ICMR. She had a great deal of interest in the project and had been participating in almost all the discussions held in connection with the project since its inception. She had worked with the ICMR Children Growth Study in 1956 and in another ICMR national project for a number of years, first as a field worker and then as a statistician. This experience was of great asset in effectively phasing the study, planning the detailed methodology, and training the field and statistical team.

The involvement of senior members of the Department of Paediatrics helped in initiating and sustaining the project as some of them later

**Figure 1.1.2:**
*From left to right: Dr S. K. Bhargava, Dr S. Ghosh, Dr V. Hooja, and Dr S. K. Sanyal. Members of Paediatric Department*

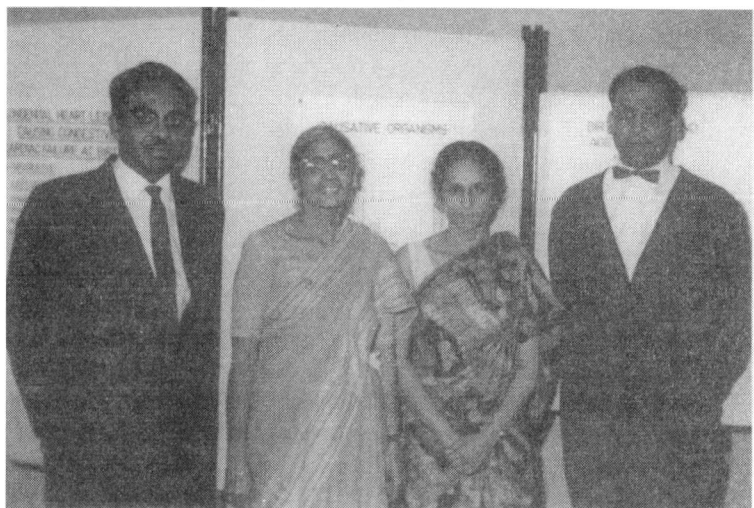

*Source:* Author.

joined the project (Figure 1.1.2). Dr V. Hooja, a paediatrician, joined the project in May 1969 as the first medical officer. As she had worked in the paediatric department, it helped in getting cooperation from the different departments of the hospital as well as from the dispensaries. The families in the project area also could derive some benefits because of her long association with the hospital. Dr S. H. Ahmed, a paediatrician, also joined the project in March 1970.

Four PHNs and one medical social worker joined in April 1969, to be followed a little later by two more PHNs. The PHNs were well trained and had some field experience.

A statistical assistant with BA in statistics was recruited towards the end of the first year (discovered accidentally at a motor garage). An assistant research officer (junior statistician) also joined in December 1969. As the work gradually increased, four more statistical assistants were appointed.

Twenty lay interviewers (all women) were appointed for fieldwork on 1 August 1969, many having higher qualifications than the required graduate degree for recruitment.

The recruitment by phasing was especially undertaken because of non-availability of adequate funds during the first year because of changes in the project objectives, methodology, and staffing pattern, revision and additional request, and receipt for supplementary grant.

The project had more unexpected trouble in store. It seemed nothing was working smoothly for any length of time for the project, and by April 1971 all our experienced PHNs decided to leave the project for better and permanent jobs in the Municipal Corporation of Delhi. It thus became necessary to change the staffing pattern and allocation of work.

Since there was a great shortage of PHNs, it became essential to select lady health visitors (LHV) for follow-up of pregnant women and recording the birth of the baby, and anthropologists/senior supervisors for recording the subsequent anthropometrics measurement of the babies.

## Training of the Staff and Standardization of Techniques

Training for all categories of staff, irrespective of the designation, was mandatory for all. In training, emphasis was laid on detailed explanations of the objectives. An elaborate key to the interviewing techniques for the various card designs was prepared and given to every member of the field staff. Each question was explained and the examples of various answers were taught. The importance of good public relations, simplicity, tact, and pleasant mannerisms was emphasized, for dealing with community and the health care providers such as midwives, general medical practitioners, and practitioners of indigenous medicine to the community. They were specially instructed to be polite and respectful and not to criticize or offer an opinion on the treatment and management of a patient by whichever medical practitioner was chosen by the family.

The PHNs and the social workers were the first to be trained. Training of the lay interviewers was more difficult. They had to be knowledgeable about some basic facts of physiology of menstruation, lactation, and pregnancy. All this took almost a month.

Another week was spent in the practice of interviewing techniques and the actual filling of the pro forma details of some patients in the hospital. It gave them practical experience and confidence and enabled us to judge their efficiency and readiness for fieldwork.

The PHNs and later the senior supervisors and anthropologists were given special training in the anthropometric techniques for measuring children and adults by Dr Darshan Singh and Dr Raghubir Singh of the anthropology department of the Delhi University. The recording of the height of women was carried out by trained anthropologists only after standardizing their techniques. PHNs and the health visitors were also trained to record blood pressure and estimate the haemoglobin content of the blood by Sahli's method.

It was decided to study the natural course of the disease and, hence, the staff was strictly instructed not to offer any advice or interfere in treatment to the family. The advice was only given when sought, or if the illness was considered severe enough to be a risk.

## Schedules/Pro Forma for the Study

For the initial phase of the study, 13 schedules were finalized. These are briefly described (Figure 1.1.3).

1. **Household Schedule:** This was mainly designed to collect the demographic information for each and every household under consideration for the study. This contained questions regarding the socio-economic status, demographics, environmental, sanitation, and total number of family members with bifurcation of number of married woman, number of children, and total family income.

2. **Individual Family Member Schedule:** This schedule was contemplated to collect the information regarding the name, sex, age, relationship to the head of the household, marital status, education, and occupation.

3. **Individual Schedule for Married Woman and their Pregnancy History:** This was designed to gather information regarding married women and their pregnancy history. This had the age, religion, education, marital status, pregnancy status, menopause, age at marriage, order of pregnancy, plurality, and last menstrual period (LMP) date.

4. **Individual Schedule for Non-pregnant Married Women:** This schedule provided information regarding the present age, number of living children, family planning practices and menstrual cycle, and two monthly rounds of registering the women for their missed period and further follow-up.

**Figure 1.1.3:**
*Schedules used for primary data collection*

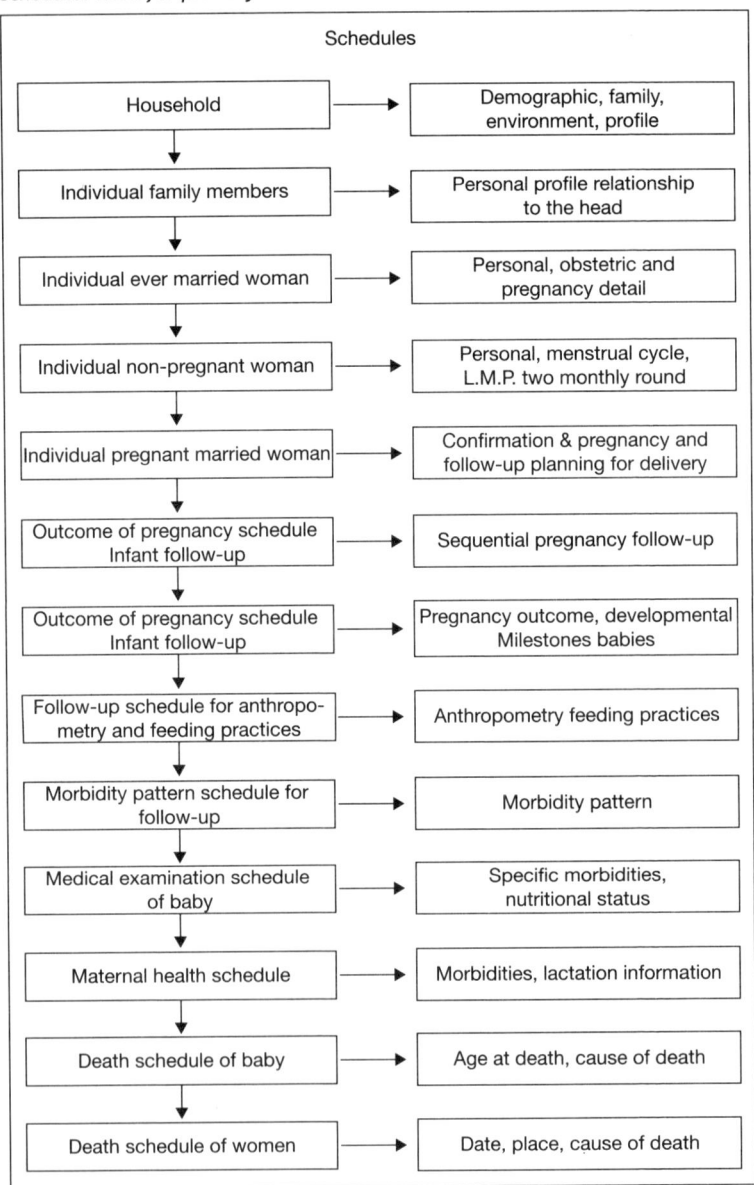

Schedules

| Household | → | Demographic, family, environment, profile |
| Individual family members | → | Personal profile relationship to the head |
| Individual ever married woman | → | Personal, obstetric and pregnancy detail |
| Individual non-pregnant woman | → | Personal, menstrual cycle, L.M.P. two monthly round |
| Individual pregnant married woman | → | Confirmation & pregnancy and follow-up planning for delivery |
| Outcome of pregnancy schedule Infant follow-up | → | Sequential pregnancy follow-up |
| Outcome of pregnancy schedule Infant follow-up | → | Pregnancy outcome, developmental Milestones babies |
| Follow-up schedule for anthropo-metry and feeding practices | → | Anthropometry feeding practices |
| Morbidity pattern schedule for follow-up | → | Morbidity pattern |
| Medical examination schedule of baby | → | Specific morbidities, nutritional status |
| Maternal health schedule | → | Morbidities, lactation information |
| Death schedule of baby | → | Age at death, cause of death |
| Death schedule of women | → | Date, place, cause of death |

*Source:* Author.

5. **Individual Schedule for Married Pregnant Women:** This was used for follow-up of pregnancy after confirmation of the conception or pregnancy. It also collected information on family planning practices, antenatal care, planning for delivery, occupation, number of living children, expected date of delivery, and type of termination of pregnancy.

6. **Pregnant Woman Follow-up Schedule:** It provided sequential follow-up of pregnant woman during the pregnancy and recorded weight gain during pregnancy and other pertinent findings at the follow-up.

7. **Outcome of Pregnancy Schedule with Follow-up of Baby for Milestone**: This schedule records the pregnancy outcome and the milestones of the baby on different follow-ups, with birth weight, congenital abnormalities, type of delivery, vaccination status, and mortality, if any, till one year of age.

8. **Baby Follow-up Schedule for Anthropometry and Feeding Practices**: In this schedule, the anthropometric measurements and feeding practices history had been recorded with each follow-up date of visit.

9. **Morbidity Pattern Schedule of Baby:** Basically, this schedule was designed to record the morbidity pattern on the follow-up, which contains the information regarding the date of visit, age at visit, and illness, if any.

10. **Medical Examination Schedule of Baby**: This schedule contains the information regarding the specific morbidities, dentition history on the date of visit, and the nutritional status of the baby.

11. **Maternal Health Schedule:** In this, the specific information about morbidities of the married woman along with the lactation information was recorded.

12. **Death Schedule of Baby:** In case of any death, then this schedule recorded the information regarding date of death, sex, date of birth, place of death, and cause of death.

13. **Death Schedule of Women:** In case of any death of a woman, then it was recorded in this schedule with information regarding date of death, type of follow-up of the woman, place of death, and cause of death.

## Planning Different Components of the Study

The entire work of the project had to be phased, and different phases were thus planned for smooth working, supervision, and monitoring.

1. **Phase One: From April 1969 to September 1969:** Selection of population, recruitment of staff and their training, and pre-testing of schedules and field technique. Period: 6 months.
2. **Phase Two: From October 1969 to May 1970:** Preliminary census of the selected area. Period: 2 months.
3. **Phase Three: From December 1969 to May 1970:** Initial round of contact with all the families in the area. Period 6 months.
4. **Phase Four: From 1 December 1969 to 30 November 1972:** Period for enrolment of cohort. Period: 3 years.

### Repeating of the Census

Every year in October and November: Once a year.

### Defining Objectives

The principle aim of the study was to determine the effect of social, environmental, biological, and related factors on the outcome of pregnancy, birth weight, gestation, foetal growth retardation, congenital malformations, physical growth, and development of the children in early life. It was expected that during the study information on knowledge, attitude, and practices in the community relating to family planning methods, immunizations, and reproductive biology and fertility would also become available. As the follow-up of pregnancy and children was predetermined and age-specific, it was also considered possible to study the nutritional status of children and growth as related to protein energy malnutrition. Accordingly, the following objectives of the study were identified during different phases of the study.

## General Objectives

1. To record the demographic pattern of an urban population in South Delhi community and to prospectively study the vital statistics such as birth rate, foetal loss rate, peri-natal, neonatal, and infant and age-specific childhood mortality rates.
2. To follow the ever-married women of childbearing age from the pre-pregnant state to the conception and the termination of the pregnancy and relate the outcome with social, environmental, and biological factors.
3. To establish the childhood growth pattern in an urban cohort.
4. To study the fertility pattern and family planning practices and their trends in the study population.

## Specific Objectives

1. **Low Birth Weight:**
   To study the problem of LBW in India with special reference to its prevalence, causes, outcome, and sequelae and relate them to birth weight, gestational age, and foetal growth retardation.
2. **Physical Growth:**
   To study early childhood growth and development pattern in cohort children and factors influencing them.
3. **Nutrition:**
   a. To study the nutritional status of the cohort children in early childhood for prevalence of protein energy malnutrition and factors contributing to its occurrence.
   b. To study age-independent indices for assessment of nutritional status of children.
4. **Congenital Malformations:**
   To study the prevalence of congenital malformation in a longitudinal follow-up of a birth cohort.
5. **Attrition and Loss to Follow-up:**
   To describe the loss to follow-up of the cohorts, the reasons for the same, and ways to contain the loss to follow-up.

# 2

# Launching of the Study

The study was launched on 1 December 1969 with the booking of individual families by the lay interviewers. This consisted of actual census of the population residing in the nine study areas of Lajpat Nagar I to IV, Harinagar Ashram, and its sub-area. This was carried out in October and November 1969. It was repeated each year to check the movement of population and to ensure the inclusion of every family. Families without an ever-married woman were excluded from this study.

## Methodology of the Study

The census of the population was followed by booking of individual families by the lay interviewers in December 1969. Complete information regarding the address, the number, names and ages (completed years), and the marital status of members of the household was recorded. Children above 14 years of age were considered as adults. Members of the household who were staying away permanently, for example, married offspring; children living in the village with their relations, etc., were excluded. On the other hand, the dependents living with the family were included. The relationship of each member of the family to the head of the household, type of family—whether nuclear or joint—occupation, income, education, type of housing, sanitation, toilet and water facilities, and independent or shared were duly recorded.

# Registration of the Ever-married Women

At the time of the initial visit, a card was made for each ever-married woman with particulars of her current marital and menstruation status, occupation, present age, age at marriage, and details of her past obstetric history. The reproductively active women were followed on a separate pro forma with details of menstrual history such as length of the cycle, regularity or otherwise, and duration of menstrual flow. The questions relating to family planning were scrupulously avoided as families shunned family planning workers. The family planning questions were deferred for later and included the acceptance, regularity, and type of the contraceptive devices used. At each visit, women who became non-eligible because of secondary amenorrhea, menopause, hysterectomy, and sterilization of the husband or the wife were excluded from the follow-up (Figure 1.2.1).

**Figure 1.2.1:**
*Registering the cohort*

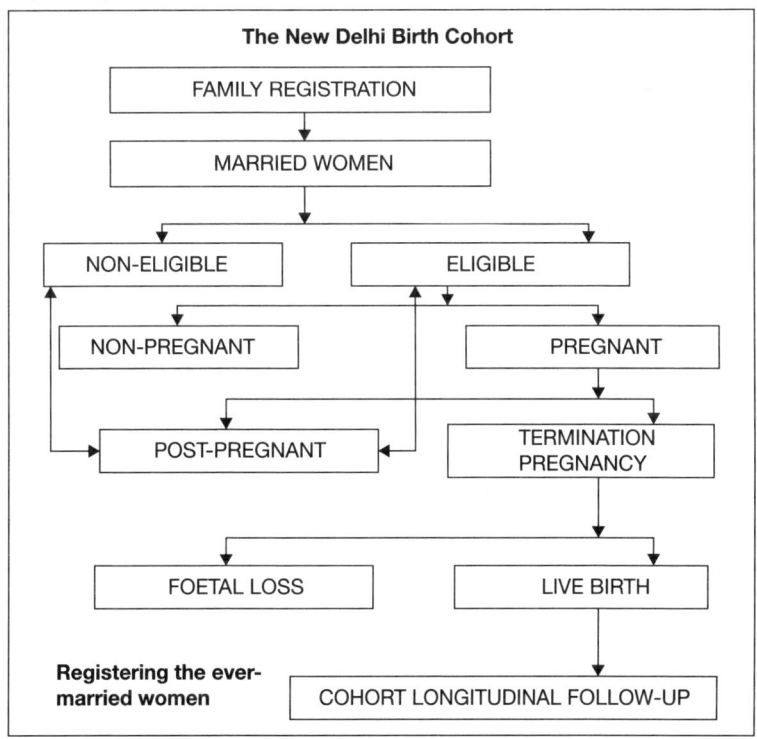

**Source:** Author.

## Pregnancy Follow-Up

### Detection and Confirmation of Pregnancy

Each subject was followed up regarding the menstrual cycle every 2 months ±3 days, and the first day of the LMP were noted. In the event of a missed menstrual period, the PHN/LHV contacted the woman within a fortnight near about the next expected period and if the woman still failed to menstruate then she was booked as a pregnant woman and followed as per protocol on pregnancy pro forma. Detailed information on whether it was a planned pregnancy or otherwise, likely place of antenatal care, and delivery was also sought.

### Pregnancy Follow-Up

The pregnant woman was followed by the PHN/LHV every 2 months +3 days, for recording illness and morbidity, such as, anaemia, urinary problems, bleeding per vagina, fever, rash, and/or any other problem. The blood pressure and haemoglobin were checked once during the third trimester. The record of antenatal visits was made and any hospitalization or use of drugs was recorded.

Nearly 2 weeks prior to the expected date of delivery, the PHN/LHV checked the weight of the pregnant woman to assess the weight gain during pregnancy and then followed her as a 'due case'. Since the objective of the study was to record the nature and type of delivery, anthropometric measurement of the newborn within 48 hours of birth, and any congenital malformations, it was considered essential to visit the household almost on alternate days from 38 weeks of pregnancy to check about the birth of the infant. We explored all possibilities by which the information regarding the birth of the infant could be immediately brought to us by the family member, either by post, mail, or telephone. But, this was not found feasible, practical, or reliable. Even stamped postcards left with the family regarding the information on birth were hardly used by them.

However, to our surprise it was found that despite frequent visits, a considerable number of birth weights were being missed as many women delivered prior to the expected date of delivery and, hence, the infants could not be reached within 48 hours of birth. The birth weight recording was therefore missed, which was one of the most important objectives and parameters of the study. We were therefore compelled to modify the methodology. The birth measurement were now expected to be taken within 72 hours of birth and the follow-up as 'due cases' was begun on the completion of 37 weeks of pregnancy rather than 38 weeks as before. Prior to the change of methodology, a pilot study was undertaken at the Safdarjung Hospital which did not show any significant difference in weight taken at 48 hours and 72 hours. At this time, the gestational age was calculated and noted down along with the parity. The type of termination, whether live birth, twin, abortion, or stillbirth, was also documented.

### Pregnancy Outcome

After termination of a pregnancy, the pregnant woman's pro forma and pregnancy follow-up pro forma were closed, and post-pregnancy pro forma was made after one week post-delivery. This also had the date, place, and type of termination as well as particulars of lochia, lactation, and any morbidity after termination.

In the post-partum period, the woman was revisited at the end of 1 month by a PHN and thereafter every 2 months ±3 days for one year by the interviewer for record of morbidity, commencement of the menstrual period, and date of first day of LMP. If she became pregnant again, the fact was noted, she was rebooked as a pregnant woman, a new set of pro formas were made for her, and the same methodology as for the earlier pregnancy was followed.

### Infant and Children Follow-Up

After birth, the infant was followed at home at the specified age of every 3 months ±1 week till the age of 2 years ±2 weeks thereafter, till the child attained adulthood by the age of 20 years.

Every child was followed for survival and physical growth till the age of 20 years. In addition, the children were followed for congenital malformations, breastfeeding and top feeding pattern, primary immunizations, milestones and CD, and nutritional status in early childhood.

## *Adult Follow-Ups*

The cohorts were periodically followed again from 1998 till date at varying ages and periods for different studies. These are described in the later chapters.

# 3

# Demography

## Physical Characteristics and Housing

In general, the area was chosen to be a mix of population, housing, environment, socio-economic status, sanitation and water supply, and related factors to provide a representative urban cohort. It was located in South Delhi in a 12 sq km area. This was well demarcated by geographic lines.

The project area was divided into nine areas for convenience of follow-up and monitoring. The population and living characteristics of each area are briefly described from an interim analysis which was later published.

The total population covered in this analysis was 113,202 in the nine areas for convenience of follow-up, monitoring, and analysis. The population in different areas varied from 4,104 to 31,045. The per capita income area wise is given in Table 1.3.1. Over 2/3rd or 76.8% of the earned income is between ₹0 and 100 per month with only 2.4% having an income of ₹300 or more (Table 1.3.1).

### Area I: Lajpat Nagar I

This was inclusive of Railway Colony and Krishna Market. The population mainly comprised the settlers who came from West Pakistan after partition of the country. These had 2,742 families with a population of 14,878. About 73% of the families were nuclear. The per capita income per month in 79.9% was between ₹0 and 100, in 17.5% between ₹101

**Table 1.3.1:**
*Area-wise per capita income*

| Area | Total Population | 0–100 n (%) | 101–200 n (%) | 201–300 n (%) | >300 n (%) |
|---|---|---|---|---|---|
| I | 14,878 (13.1%) | 11,893 (79.9) | 2,553 (17.2) | 276 (1.8) | 156 (1.1) |
| II | 13,907 (12.2%) | 9,669 (69.5) | 3,092 (22.2) | 777 (5.6) | 369 (2.7) |
| III | 4,104 (3.6%) | 1,116 (27.2) | 1,513 (36.9) | 722 (17.6) | 753 (18.3) |
| IV | 31,045 (27.4%) | 21,881 (70.5) | 6,669 (21.5) | 1,831 (5.9) | 664 (2.1) |
| V | 4,441 (3.9%) | 4,275 (96.3) | 159 (3.6) | 5 (0.1) | 2 (0.04) |
| VI | 11,734 (10.3%) | 10,300 (87.8) | 1,314 (11.2) | 98 (0.8) | 22 (0.2) |
| VII | 13,539 (11.9%) | 9,383 (69.3) | 2,686 (19.8) | 754 (5.6) | 716 (5.3) |
| VIII | 8,739 (7.7%) | 8,068 (92.3) | 550 (6.3) | 108 (1.2) | 13 (0.2) |
| IX | 10,815 (9.5%) | 10,409 (96.3) | 338 (3.1) | 59 (0.6) | 9 (0.08) |
| Total | 113,202 | 86,994 (76.8) | 18,874 (16.7) | 4,630 (4.1) | 2,704 (2.4) |

*Source:* Author.

and 200, and in 2.9% above ₹200. More than 50% lived in two-room accommodations, with 36.5% in one room and 11.4% in three rooms or more. The average number of person living per room was three.

## Area II: Lajpat Nagar II

This included Central Market, Pushpa Market, and Vinoba Puri. The population was mostly settlers from West Pakistan. This had 2,702 families with a population of 13,907 who had small self-owned business or were in service. Almost 75% were nuclear families. About 69.5% had a per capita per month income of ₹100 or less, 22.2% between ₹101 and 200, 5.59% between ₹201 and 300, and 2.6% ₹300 more. About 36.3% lived in a single room, 44.0% in two rooms, and the remaining in three or more room accommodation. About 2.6 people lived per room.

## Area III: Lajpat Nagar III

It comprised part of Ring Road, Feroz Gandhi Road, and part of Link Road. It had the lowest mixed population of 4,104 with 834 families, with 70% of them being nuclear families. Approximately 27.1% had a per capita per month income of ₹0–100, 36.8% between ₹101 and 200,

17.5% between ₹201 and 300, and 18.3% had an income of ₹300 or more. About 1.8 people lived per room. It had bungalows, kothis, own businesses, and shops. It was relatively richer area of the population

### Area IV: Lajpat Nagar IV

This had several colonies with mixed heterogeneous population in colonies such as old and new double storey, Amar colony, Dayanand Colony, Guru Nanak Market and a part of ring road, Sant Nagar, Ghari, Prakash Mohalla, and Amritpuri. It had population of 31,045 with 6,237 families. Of these, 70.7% earned between ₹0 and 100 per person per month, 21.48% between ₹100 and 200, 5.9% between ₹201 and 300, and only 2.1% above ₹300. Half the population lived in two-bedroom accommodations, 41.6% in one room and the remaining in three or more rooms. An average of 2.9 persons lived in one room. Most of the population owned the houses or paid a small rent.

### Area V: Nehru Nagar

This was a small colony with 803 families and a population of only 441 people. Almost all (96.2%) earned a per capita per month income of ₹0–100, 3.5% had a per capita/per month income of ₹101–200, and few had over ₹200. These were mostly *pucca* (concrete) double-storey houses, with 85% living in one room, 14.1% in two rooms, and less than 1% in three rooms or more. About 4–5 people lived per room. The population consisted mainly of service people or petty shopkeepers.

### Area VI: Srinivaspuri

This part of the project area mainly consisted of government quarters along with a private colony and some unauthorized construction. It had 2,294 families, with about 60% being nuclear, and a population of 11,374. About 87.8% had a per capita per month income of ₹0–100, 11.1% had an income between ₹101 and 200, and remaining had above ₹200 per person per month; 67.2% lived in one room, 31.1% in two rooms, and 1.61% in three rooms or more with the average occupancy per room being 3.8 persons.

## Area VII: Jangpura A, Jangpura B, Jangpura Extension, and Pant Nagar

This is one of the posh areas of the Delhi. It had a mixed population including businessmen and high government officials. The population was 15,539 with 2,659 families and with 76.9% being nuclear. About 9.1% earned between ₹0 and 100 per person per month, 19.8% between ₹101 and 200, and almost 5% each above 200 and 300 per person per month. About 34.0% lived in one room, 42.8% in two, and 8.1% in a three or more room accommodation. The average occupancy per room was 2.5 people.

## Area VIII: Bhogal

It had 1,649 families with an overwhelming 82% being nuclear. The per capita per month income in over 90% of them was ₹0–100, 6.2% earned between ₹101 and 200, and remaining few above ₹200. It had cluster of havelis with single-room accommodations. About 63.5% lived in one room, 28.2% in two, and 8.1% in three rooms or more. The average occupancy per room was 3.6 persons.

## Area IX: Hari Nagar Ashram

This had four colonies, namely, Bhagwan Nagar, Jiwan Nagar, Siddarth Basti, and Sunlight Colony I and II. These areas had a mix population with service people, self-employed auto rickshaw drivers, and others. It had a population of 10,815 with 2,202 families of which 88.5% were nuclear. Almost all or 96.0% had a per capita per month income of ₹0–100, 6.2% had between ₹101 and 200, and very few had above ₹200. About 83.8% resided in one room, 12.5 in two rooms and 3.5% in three or more rooms. The average occupancy in a room was 4 persons (Figure 1.3.1).

## Population Characteristics

The project was located in a well-demarcated 12 sq km area in South Delhi. It had a population of 119,799 of which 61,698 (51.5%) were males and 58,089 (48.5%) were females. About 49.4% were children

**Figure 1.3.1:**
*Distribution of families according to number of rooms in different areas*

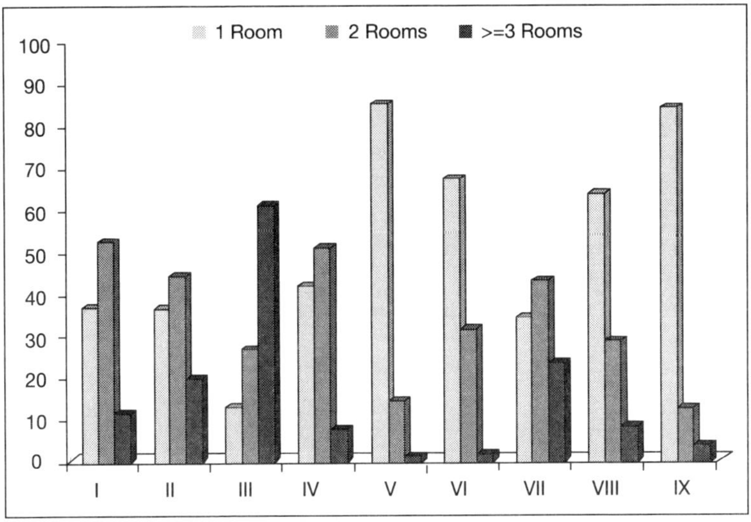

*Source:* Author.

up to 19 years of age. Hindus, with 82.8% of the population, were the predominant community followed by Sikhs 13.1%, Christians 2.1%, Muslims 1.9%, Jains 0.6%, and the remaining other communities.

In the selected population, 95.1% of the heads of the families were married, 3.7% widowed, 0.01% divorced, and 0.09% separated from their spouses. Majority of the population had been married only once.

Only 8.5% of families were original natives of Delhi. Most of the population (50.7%) had migrated from West Pakistan after Partition and had settled in this area. The migrants from other states included Uttar Pradesh (16.2%), Punjab (11.1%), Haryana (2.1%), and from Rajasthan, Tamil Nadu, and Kerala (1–2%). About 8.5% of the families were living here since birth and the majority (46.5%) were residing in the project area for more than 20 years. Only 6.6% had been living there for less than a year.

The per capita monthly income of ₹0–100 was recorded for 60.2%, ₹101–200 for 26.3%, ₹201–300 for 8.2% and only 5.3% had income above ₹300 or more per month. The mean per capita income per month was ₹106.

About 5.8% of the population lived in government quarters, 44.7% in self-owned accommodation, and 48.3% in rented accommodation. Less than 2% lived in other kind of accommodation.

Protected water supply was received by 81.9% of the families. Of these, 48% had an independent supply and the others had a shared water supply. About 12.7% of the families received unprotected water with almost all getting it from a shared source. About 5.4% of the families received both protected and unprotected water supply.

The sanitation conditions showed 53% with flush kind of latrines. Amongst these, 30% had independent and 23% had shared facility. Scavenger cleaned toilets were used by a high 1/3 or 31.1% of the families. In these, 6.8% had unshared and 24.3% had shared facility. The open field was used by as many as 14.2% and the pit kind of toilet by 1.7% of the families.

About 90% of the head of the households were educated, and only 8.2% were illiterate. Around 29.7% received education up to middle class, 30.5% matric, and 31.4% up to college level. The male literacy level showed 6.2% as illiterates, 26.1% with primary and middle class education, 35.9% as matriculates, and 31.6% as having received college education. In comparison, the female literacy showed 24.0% to be as illiterate, 34.2% with primary and middle class, 24.3% as matriculates, and 17.3% with college education.

Only 43.7% of in the family had regular employment. They had trained in different kinds of occupations. These varied from being salesmen (10.8%), clerical or related work (9.6%), professional/technical personnel (8.6%), craftsmen and weavers (4.14%), drivers and conductors and allied types (3.6%), and administrators and executives, compositors and printers, and waiters and recreation workers (about 2% each). About 33.3% were housewives. The remaining population included 23.2% unemployed students and retired and old persons.

## Profile of the Ever-married Women

The study had 25,708 ever-married women. The age distribution being 14–19 years (4.3%), 20–30 years (37.3%), 31–40 years (30.3%), 40–49 years (14.8%), and the remaining were above 49 years of age. Amongst these women, 4,484 (17.4%) had menopause and 2,381 (9.2%) were either divorced, separated, or widow.

Most of the women were low or low middle-income group. The per capita per month income distribution was ₹0–50/ in 24.7%, ₹51–100/ in 35.4%, ₹100–200 in 26.7%, and 13.0% with an income of ₹201 and more. Most of the women were literates. About 60% of these were middle class or matriculates and 12.6% had college education. The illiterates were 27.4%.

## Fertility

Fertility was assessed by the number of pregnancies. In the reproductive period of 13–49 years, teenage marriages were very common. In the 25,708 women, 18,931 (73.6%) were below 19 years of age. Of these, 5,249 (20.4%) were 14 years or less and 13,682 (53.2%) were between 15 and 19 years of age. These women had a fertility period of 20–30 years or more. In 10.6% of the women, no pregnancies were recorded. About 1/3rd (29.0%) had 1–2, 38–48% had 3–4 and almost 1/5th or 21.7% had five or more pregnancies. The mean number of pregnancies was 3.16.

## Age at Marriage

An early marriage seemed to be the norm in those days. About 18,931 (73.6%) got married in their teens by 19 years of age. Amongst these, as many as 5,249 (20.4%) had married by 14 years of age. A quarter or 25.1% married between 20 and 30 years of age and few beyond it.

Education directly influenced the age of marriage. In women marrying by 14 years of age, 42.8% were illiterates as compared to only 4.1% being matriculates and above. In contrast, 77.3% of the college educated married after 19 years of age. The mean age at marriage increased directly with an increase in education level.

A pattern similar to education was seen with the income of the family. The mean age at marriage increased from 14.7 years with per capita income of less than ₹20 per month to 17.7 years with per capita income of ₹51–100 per and to 20.15% with per capita income of more than ₹200 per month (Table 1.3.2).

Education seemed to play a stronger role in the determination of age at marriage. College educated women with an income of ₹50 per capita per month had a mean age of 20.45 years as compared to 16.5 years in illiterates with per capita of over ₹200 per month.

In all religions, majority of women got married between 15 and 19 years of age. Muslims had larger number of marriage at 14 years or less as compared to Hindus, Sikhs, Jains, and Christians. The mean age at

**Table 1.3.2:**
*Mean age at marriage by per capita income and literacy*

| Per capita income (in ₹.) | Literacy | | | | | | | | | | | | | |
|---|---|---|---|---|---|---|---|---|---|---|---|---|---|---|
| | Illiterate | | Literate | | Primary | | Middle | | Matric | | College | | Total | |
| | N | Mean | N | Mean | N | Mean | N | Mean | N | Mean | N | Mean | N | Mean |
| 0–100 | 6,492 | 14.67 | 1208 | 15.39 | 3,772 | 16.97 | 3,261 | 17.16 | 2,671 | 19.14 | 676 | 20.87 | 18,080 | 16.54 |
| 101–200 | 436 | 15.25 | 262 | 15.89 | 576 | 16.34 | 767 | 17.52 | 1,858 | 19.78 | 1,227 | 21.51 | 5,126 | 18.89 |
| >200 | 66 | 16.50 | 64 | 16.55 | 145 | 16.63 | 186 | 16.94 | 629 | 19.93 | 1,335 | 28.80 | 2,425 | 24.20 |
| Total | 6,994 | 14.72 | 1,534 | 15.52 | 4,493 | 16.88 | 4,214 | 17.22 | 5,158 | 19.47 | 3,238 | 24.38 | 25,631 | 17.74 |

*Source:* Author.

marriage for Muslims was 16.24 as compared to other communities which varied between 17.1 and 18.1 years.

## Consummation of Marriage

In an overwhelming numbers of 86.6%, the consummation of marriage was effected within one year of marriage. In women marrying 14 years of age or before, cohabitation was recorded later than the marriages which happened after 14 years of age. The duration between marriage and its consummation decreased with an increase in age at marriage. It was 1.6 years at 14 years of age, 0.13 between 15 and 19 years, and 0.02 at 24 years of age and above. This may be due to the practice of *Gauna*, which is a northern Indian custom, and the ceremony is associated with the consummation of marriage in the community.

Cohabitation started early in educated women. In illiterates, 65.7% had consummation within one year as compared to 90–100% in those educated from primary to college level. The mean duration varied from 1.13 years in illiterates to 0.04 in matriculates and 0.01 in collegiate. The economic status or income showed a linear correlation with consummation period, and it decreased from 1.1 years in per capita income of less than ₹20 per month to 0.1 years in income of ₹201 per month. The literacy and per capita income affected the duration between marriage and consummation independent of each other. Religion did not show a striking pattern and did not seem to influence the consummation of marriage.

About 40% of the women had their first child within 2 years of consummation of marriage. Educated mothers seemed to attain motherhood earlier than less educated or illiterates. Thus majority of matriculates and graduates (55%) had their first child within first 2 years of marriage as compared to only 25.8% in those less educated.

## Age at First Pregnancy

Almost 50% of the women had teenage pregnancies, with 48.49% becoming pregnant between 15 and 19 years of age. Another 48.5% became pregnant between the optimal age of 20 and 30 years. Surprisingly, 2,404 (9.3%) women were not aware of the age when they became pregnant.

Almost four times or 63.8% of the women who had their first pregnancy in teenage were illiterates as compared to only 11.9% of graduate women of the same age. Education influencing the age at first pregnancy is seen in the findings that 84.8% of collegiate becoming pregnant at the ideal age of 20–30 years as compared to 35.1% in illiterates.

In early marriage, the interval between effective marriage and first birth is greater than in the case of late marriage. This is partly due to the fact that below 20 years of age fecundity fluctuates and is subject to have what is known as adolescent sterility with a number of anovulatory cycles. The fecundity of women is much lower before the age of 20 years than afterwards. In the present study, fertility period appeared to be the same in the women with age at marriage less than 15 years and those married between 15 and 19 years and 20 and 24 years.

Beyond 24 years, fertility period showed a gradual downward trend. This has important relevance in the debate on the minimum age of marriage. The minimum legal age of marriage in India till recently was 15, and has been recently raised to 18 years.

It has been generally acknowledged, and is also noted in the present study, that the age at marriage may make a difference to fertility if it is above 20 years of age. If fertility remains uncontrolled, the critical age beyond which marriage will really have direct impact and produce demonstrable demographic affect would be about 25 years. This has been supported by other studies [25–27, 29]. Both increased income and higher education have shown a definite influence in decreasing the number of pregnancies but literacy seems to have far more effect than income. The influence of wives' education on decreasing fertility rate has been reported in other studies [30].

### Pregnancy Status

About 60% of the women in age group of 15–20 years enjoyed a married life of more than 20 years as compared to the other age groups which varied from 14 years or less to higher age groups.

About 10.6% of the women did not have any pregnancy. The current practices of only 1–2 children was seen in 29.0%, 38–48% had 3 or 4 children, and 21.7% had 5 or more pregnancies with almost 25% amongst having 6 or more children. The mean number of pregnancies was 3.56.

Literacy did not seem to have an influence on fertility period up 8 years. The mean number of pregnancies remained almost the same in illiterates, primary to middle class, matriculates, and graduates. However, after 8 years of the fertility period, higher education especially in collegiate significantly decreased the mean number of pregnancies. The per capita income followed a pattern similar to education. Religion did not seem to influence the number of pregnancies in this study with the mean number of pregnancies in Hindus being 3.6, Sikhs 3.7, Jains 3.3, Christians 3.3, and Muslims had a lower mean of 2.7 pregnancies.

A foetal loss or a child death directly influenced the mean number of pregnancies. Thus, the mean number of pregnancies increased from 3.43 with no child death to 4.8 with one, 6.27 with two, 8.3 with four, and 10.3 with six or more child deaths. A similar progressively increasing mean number of pregnancies was seen with foetal death or abortions.

The number of living male children did not seem to influence the mean number of pregnancies, and these progressively increased from 3.74 with no male child to 9.4 or more with living male children.

## Spacing

Spacing between consecutive orders of birth is a useful index of fertility condition. The mean spacing interval between two pregnancies was 2.6 years. A large number (45.2%) of the women had children within 2 years. Neither the education level nor the age at consummation of marriage seemed to influence the birthing interval. In comparison, an increase in per capita income seemed to increase the interval between two successive pregnancies. Thus, it was 2.37 in the income group of ₹20 months and increased to 2.63 with an income between ₹51 and 100 and to 2.9 with an income of ₹200 or more. All major religions recorded almost the same spacing interval between 2.26 and 2.61 with Jains having the lowest and Hindus the highest interval level. Foetal and child death decreased the birthing interval. The death of a male child did not influence the birthing interval.

Pregnancy outcome was noted to influence the spacing between pregnancies. A linear relationship of decreased spacing interval and number of pregnancies was noted with an increase in childhood mortality and pregnancy wastages. Child survival with number of living children also recorded a similar relationship but the difference was less marked (Figure 1.3.2).

**Figure 1.3.2:**
*Depicting linear relationship between numbers of foetal loss/child death by mean number of pregnancies*

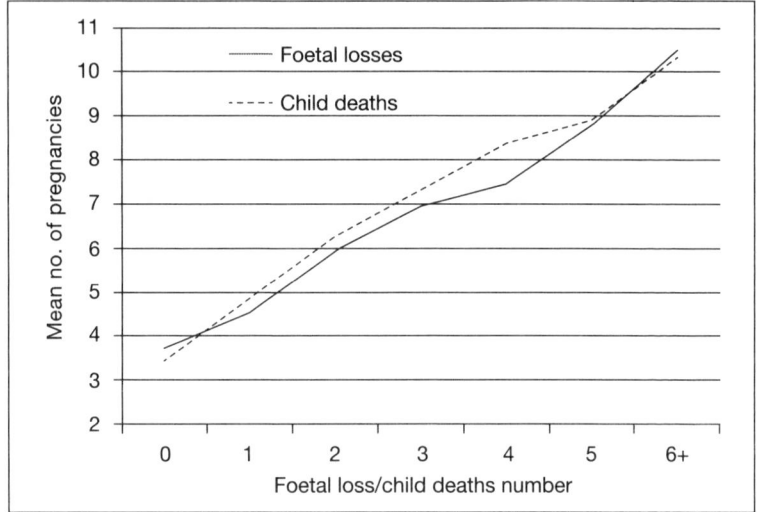

*Source:* Author.

In this study, the age at marriage had showed an inverse relationship with the number of pregnancies and consummation of marriage. An early marriage despite the risk of late occurrence of pregnancy still showed the women to have increased chances of more number of pregnancies. Literacy and per capita income seemed to inversely influence the number of pregnancies and age at marriage. It showed that the higher the age at marriage and higher the education the lesser the number of pregnancies. Women who married after 19 years of age, and were matriculates and graduates in education, had lesser number of pregnancies.

Up to 8 years of fertility period, spacing did not differ between illiterate and educated women, though economically better-off women had some influence in spacing. After the 8-year period, the spacing rate did not show a consistent relationship to literacy or economic status.

In the present study, spacing seems to be affected only by foetal loss and childhood mortality. This is understandable in view of the family wanting to have live children. However, the spacing rate was also not influenced by number of live children. This indicates a lack of motivation to limit the family, even when the family had many live children. With increase in educational level of mother and per capita income, there is little tendency towards increased spacing. Increase in age affected spacing marginally. Our results suggested that the spacing in the population under study was unaffected by such factors as socio-economic state and education and that the marginal increase in the spacing obtained in mothers of advancing age was due to natural lowering of fertility rather than other factors.

## Family Planning Practices in the Population

In the 1960s and the 1970s, when the study was planned and initiated, family planning was one of the key components of the Maternal and Child Health National Programme.

At the first contact in the 25,708 ever-married women, 16,130 (2.7%) were non-pregnant and reproductively active. Amongst these, 5,090 (31.5%) or about 1/3rd were using contraceptive methods for family planning. For about 7.9%, either of the partners was sterilized and the remaining 9,757 (60.4%) were not using any family planning method. More women were sterilized by tubectomy (714) as compared to males by vasectomy (569).

## Factors Influencing Family Planning

### Age

The numbers of users of contraceptive method increased up to 35 years of age, rising almost 10 times from 4.1% at 15 years or less to 40.5% in 26–35 years of age. It then fell to 26.5% in 36–45 years and to 6.1% in above 46 years. Sterilization was noted to be highest in 36–45 years of age (Figure 1.3.3).

### Income and Education

The increase in per capita income showed a direct relationship to acceptance of family planning. It increased from 19.2% in the lowest income of

**Figure 1.3.3:**
*Distribution by age and family planning status*

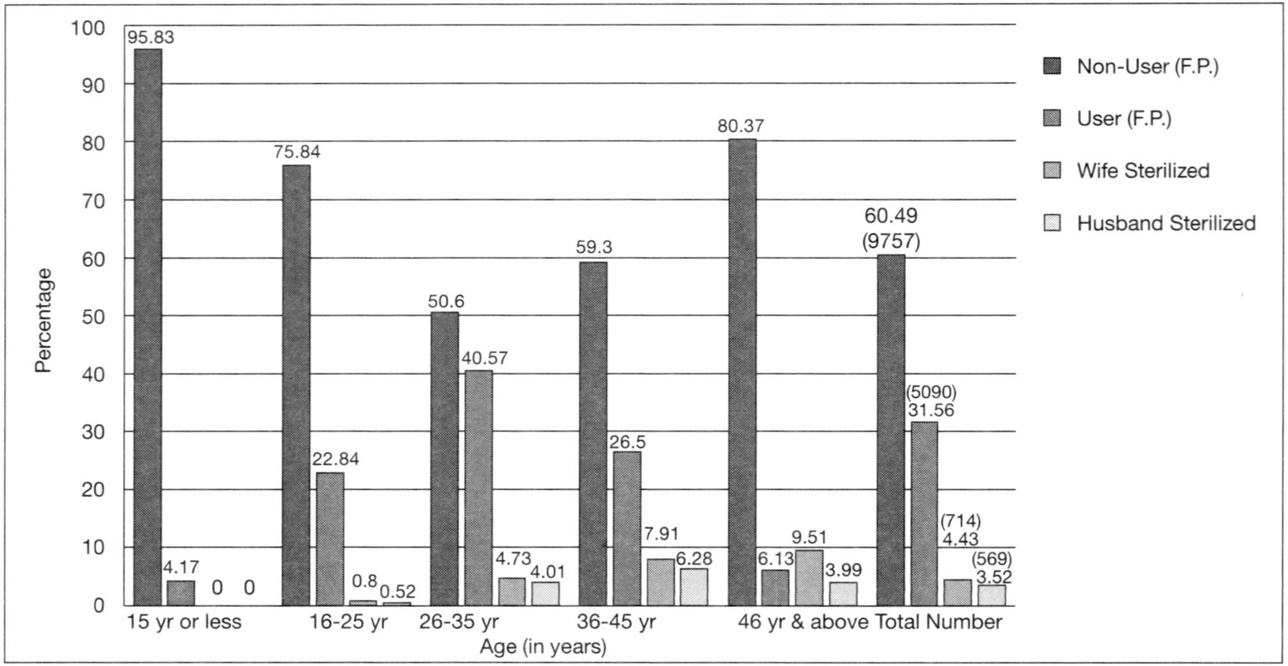

*Source:* Author.

₹20 per month to almost twice (36.2%) in the income over ₹200–300 per month, and then showed a fall in higher income. A reverse trend is seen in non-users and those opting for sterilization. The educational status recorded a trend similar to increasing income with increasing acceptance of the family planning with an increase in educational status. However, sterilization was preferred more frequently by illiterate women as compared to literate women.

## Number of Pregnancies

The number of pregnancies in users and non-users of family planning methods revealed an interesting pattern. The number of pregnancies in non-users varied from 50.9% to 72.4%. In comparison, strikingly, the number of pregnancies did not go beyond 40% in users of contraceptives. In the sterilized group, the number varied from 0.48 to 17.3% (Figure 1.3.4). Thus, it seems that the adoption of family planning methods enables a family to limit the size of their families, and with fewer members to support, it is likely to save family resources including income. This in turn may result in the availability of more economic resources to the family to improve the quality of their lives with better living conditions in housing and health, nutrition, and education of their children.

The death of one or more children seemed to adversely influence the practice of family planning. Thus, in families with no sibling deaths, the number of non-users of family planning method drop in couples with no children from 98.2% to 70.6% in couples with one, 53.6% with two, and 46.7% with four living children.

In contrast, for any given number of living children, the number of non-users rises with increase in the number of sibling death. In families with one child alive, the number of non-users rise from 70.9% with no deaths to 96.2% with four death, with two children alive the number of non-users rise from 54% with no death to 79% and with four deaths, and with four children alive from 47.9% with no death to 67.6% (Figure 1.3.5).

In contrast to child mortality, the increase in number of living children increased the acceptance of contraceptive methods. The number of contraceptive users increased from 1.8% in childless couples to 70.2% with one and about 50% with two or more living children.

**Figure 1.3.4:**
*Family planning practices and number of pregnancies*

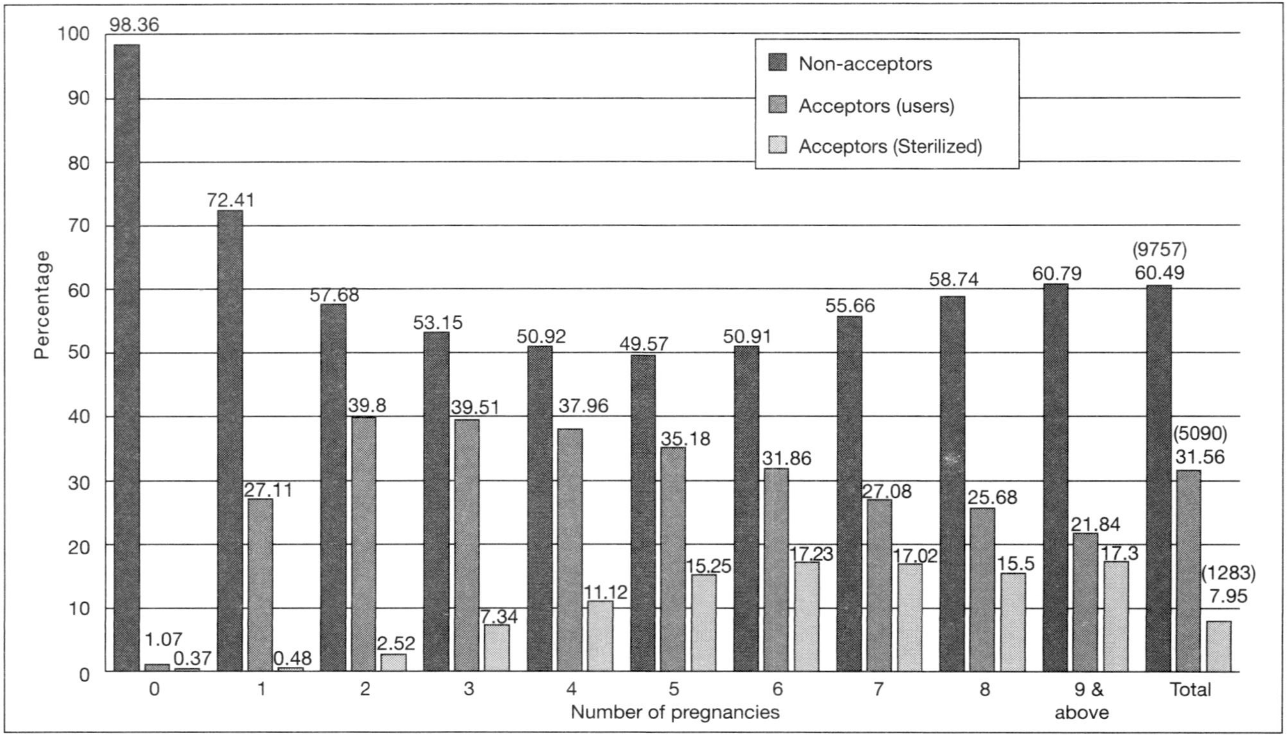

**Source:** Author.

**Figure 1.3.5:**
*Showing a direct increase in non-users of contraceptives with increase in child mortality experience*

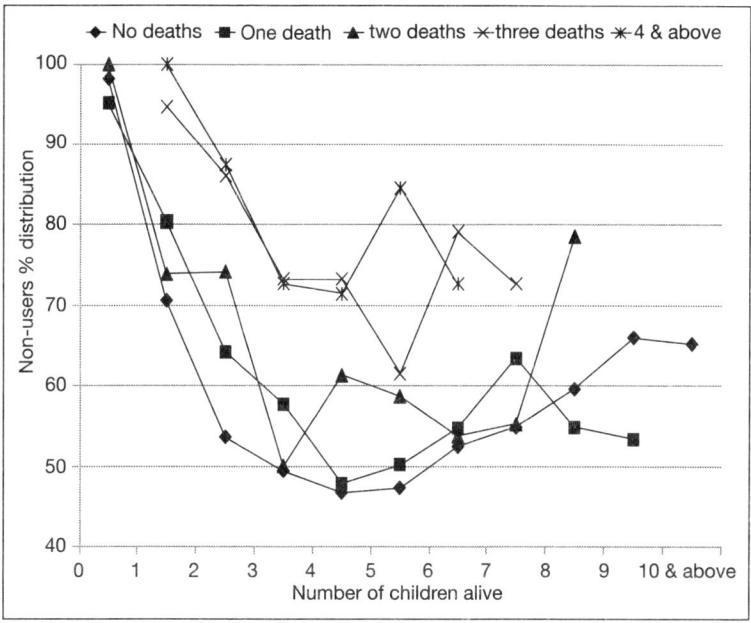

*Source:* Author.

PART 2

# The Cohort

# 1

# Pregnancy

## General Profile

There were 25,708 ever-married eligible women. Of these, 9,509 women became pregnant during the study period of 3 years and 9 months (1 April 1969–31 December 1973). Out of these, 340 cases were excluded as these had shifted out of the study area and their outcome was not known. Thus, a total of 9,169 pregnant women were followed for recording the outcome of pregnancy.

## Follow-Up

The pregnant women were followed by the PHN/LHV every 2 months +3 days for recording illness and morbidity, such as anaemia, urinary symptoms, bleeding per vaginum, fever, rash, and/or any other problem. The blood pressure and haemoglobin were checked once during the third trimester. The record of antenatal visits was made and any hospitalization or use of drugs was also noted. Nearly two weeks prior to the expected date of delivery, the PHN/LHV checked the weight of the pregnant woman to assess the weight gain during pregnancy and then followed her as 'due case'.

## Pregnancy Profile

Most of the women belonged to the low or middle-income group with 90% of the mother's family earning an income of less than ₹100 per month. Only 7.2% earned an income of more than ₹200 per month. Illiteracy was common with almost 1/3rd or about 30% of the expectant mothers being illiterate and about 40% educated until middle or matriculate. The remaining had primary education (15.4%) or were graduates (13.2%). Teenage marriages were uncommon, and only 8.3% were 19 years or less. About 70% of the mothers were in the optimal childbearing age between 20 and 30 years. Elderly expectants mothers of age 40 years or more were negligible (0.9%) and 1/5th or 20% were between 31 and 39 years of age. Majority (60%) of the women were 2–5 gravida, 13% were six gravida, or more and only 13.2% were first time pregnancies.

Pregnancy was recorded within 1 year of the last pregnancy and/or consummation of marriage in 18% of the women. However, majority of women became pregnant between 1 and 2 years of consummation of marriage and about 30% between 2 and 5 years. It was uncommon to have pregnancies after 6 years of consummation of marriage. History of past foetal deaths or losses was documented in only 13% (Table 2.1.1).

## Antenatal Care

Antenatal registration was good (76.5%) and the expectant mothers were aware of the need to register the pregnancies. But, in general, the antenatal care visits throughout the pregnancy were unsatisfactory. The pattern was almost similar in all the three trimesters and seemed to decrease with each trimester. In the multipara women, the antenatal visits increased from one visit to four or more in the first to third trimester. But even in the third trimester, only 52.4% visited only once for antenatal check-up. The antenatal care visits appeared was related to the income and education of the pregnant women and their husbands. Primipara appeared more concerned and had more number of antenatal clinic visits as compared to multipara women.

**Table 2.1.1**
*Profile of pregnant women*

| Parameter | Number | Percentage |
|---|---|---|
| Gravida | | |
| 1 | 2,169 | 27 |
| 2 to 5 | 4,818 | 60.1 |
| 6+ | 1,039 | 13 |
| **Foetal losses** | | |
| 0 | 8,277 | 87 |
| 1 to 3 | 1,185 | 12.5 |
| 4+ | 47 | 0.5 |
| **Age of mother (years)** | | |
| >19 | 664 | 8.3 |
| 20–29 | 5,701 | 71.4 |
| 30–39 | 1,546 | 19.4 |
| 40+ | 73 | 0.9 |
| **No. of years since termination of last pregnancy** | | |
| ≤1 | 1,183 | 18 |
| 1 to 2 | 3,669 | 55.8 |
| 3 to 5 | 1,363 | 20.7 |
| 6 to 10 | 358 | 5.4 |
| **Education status** | | |
| Illiterate | 2,456 | 28.8 |
| Primary | 1,310 | 15.4 |
| Middle-matric | 3,391 | 32 |
| Matric | 1,979 | 23.2 |
| College | 1,123 | 13.2 |
| **Per capita income (₹/month)** | | |
| ≤50 | 3,501 | 41 |
| 51–200 | 4,421 | 51.8 |
| 201+ | 616 | 7.2 |

*Source:* Author.

## Delivery

Of the 9,165 pregnancies, known abortions occurred in 793 and still-births in 191 (2.09%). Majority of the women planned for their deliveries and had pre-decided about the place of the delivery. Almost 70% of the cases or more delivered as per the plan. Institutional- or facility-based delivery was recorded in 64.06%. Home delivery was common (nearly 30%) and, amongst these, 93.4% of women had normal deliveries. The hospital births had higher occurrence for the need of assisted births, which was almost four times (8.45%) more frequent as compared to home deliveries (2.04%). Caesarean section was performed in only 2.3%, assisted forceps in 2.7%, and breech delivery in only 0.9% cases.

# 2

# Birth and Outcome of Cohort

## The Birth of the Cohort

The cohorts were born at different places which included their homes, government and private hospitals, maternity and child welfare centres, and nursing homes in Delhi. An effort was made to reach each cohort as soon as possible, within 72 hours of births, to record their birth history and measurements.

## The Newborn

A total of 8,181 births were recorded for the study. These newborn infants constituted what is now known as 'the NDBC' (Figure 2.2.1). In the 8,181 cohorts, 8,030 were single birth and 151 multiple births. In the 75 multiple births, 74 were twins and one had triplets. In single births, males (52.04%) were more.

## Definitions and Terms Used

The live births in medical or even in lay terms are called or defined by the time they spend in womb or in the uterus.

**Figure 2.2.1:**
*Logo of the NDBC*

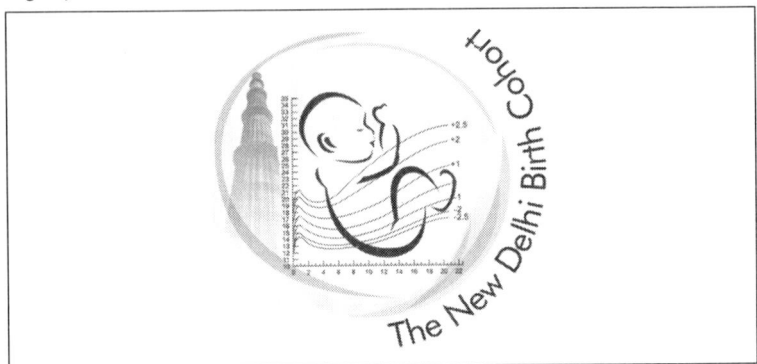

*Source:* Author.

**Gestation:** The time between missing the first day of the LMP and the date of birth of the infant in completed weeks is called the gestational age or period of gestation. It is always calculated in completed weeks. It is also called the intrauterine period and the period of foetal or baby growth in uterus. A normal period of gestation or intrauterine period is nine months or 40 weeks or 280 days.

**Preterm:** The gestational age or the period of gestation or intrauterine period has always been used medically to define the babies as preterm if the infant is born early or before 37 weeks of gestation period.

**Term:** A term infant refers to a gestational age between 37 and 41 weeks.

**Post-term:** A post-term infant refers to a gestational age of 42 weeks or more.

## Period of Gestation or Gestational Age

In the NDBC, the gestational age was correctly known in 7,085 infants of the cohort. Of these 7,085 infants, 71.6% of them were term, 16.4% were preterm, and 12.4% were post-term infants. This birthing pattern was more or less consistent with what was seen generally in the country.

## Preterm

The prevalence of preterm births across the globe varies from 5% to 18%. About 22.5 million of these are born annually and almost 1 million of these premature infants are believed to die. The survivors have the potential risk of a lifelong disability in cognitive functions, motor and physical deficits, and learning, visual, and hearing deficits. India is the biggest contributor to the global burden of premature births and population. The prematurity prevalence in India is reported to vary from 5% to 22%.

In the NDBC the prevalence of preterm births was 16.4%. Amongst these preterm births, 5.01% delivered at gestation of 28 weeks or less and 11.03 between 29 and 36 weeks. The infants delivering at 36 weeks were 5.2% or almost 2/3rd of all preterm infants (Figure 2.2.2 and Table 2.2.1).

One of the most significant findings is the pattern of the occurrence of preterm births at different gestations between 28 and 36 weeks of gestation. 1/3rd of preterm births occur at 36 weeks and there is an urgent

**Figure 2.2.2:**
*Comparison of distribution of births at different gestation in NDBC and the USA*

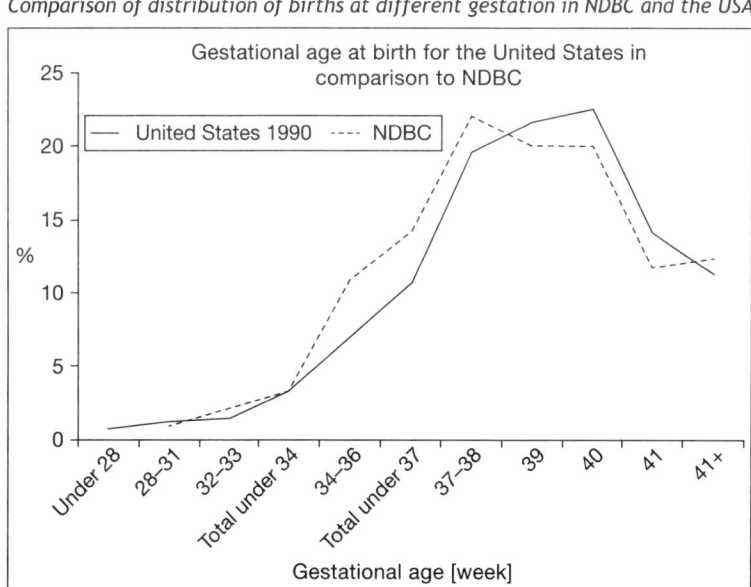

**Source:** National Vital Statistics Reports. Vol. 64, No. 1, 15 January 2015.

**Table 2.2.1:**
*Gestation distribution from 30 weeks to 42+ weeks in cohort subjects*

| Gestation (weeks) | N | Percentage (%) |
|---|---|---|
| 30 | 20 | 0.3 |
| 31 | 43 | 0.7 |
| 32 | 53 | 0.9 |
| 33 | 83 | 1.4 |
| 34 | 144 | 2.4 |
| 35 | 200 | 3.3 |
| 36 | 315 | 5.2 |
| 37 | 475 | 7.8 |
| 38 | 860 | 14.2 |
| 39 | 1,208 | 20 |
| 40 | 1,187 | 20 |
| 41 | 712 | 11.8 |
| 42± | 751 | 12.4 |
| **Total** | **6,051** | |

*Source:* Author.

need to epidemiologically investigate this phenomenon. The maximum births are occurring at 37–38 weeks of gestation. This is at variance with the birthing pattern from the developed world and is similar to what has been reported later in other Indian studies [28,36]. A successful intervention at this gestational age to affect a shift of the gravidogram or the gestation curve to the right by only one week will decrease the burden of preterm to almost half of the current prevalence. This shift will make the prevalence of preterm in India comparable to the developed countries.

Numerous factors are believed to contribute to causation of preterm births, either directly or by predisposing to it. In the NDBC environment, the type of housing, per capita income, maternal education, primi parity, maternal age of 35 years or more, age at marriage, antenatal care, and place of delivery were associated with preterm birth. Amongst the specific factors, poor environment such as non-flush latrines, poor socioeconomic status, illiteracy, poor antenatal care, and home delivery were significant contributory factors ($p < .001$) for preterm births (Table 2.2.2 and Figure 2.2.3).

**Table 2.2.2:**
*Factors influencing gestational age in cohort subjects*

| | Gestation (weeks) | | |
| | Preterm Gestation <37 weeks | Term Preterm Gestation ≥37–41 weeks | |
| | % (n) | % (n) | P value |
|---|---|---|---|
| Latrine facility | | | |
| Shared | 78.9 (758) | 72.8 (3,579) | <0.001 |
| Not shared | 21.1 (203) | 27.2 (1,334) | |
| Type of latrine | | | |
| Flush | 32.9 (316) | 41.0 (2,016) | |
| Pit | 3.1 (30) | 1.4 (69) | <0.001 |
| Scavenger cleaned | 37.3 (358) | 38.9 (1,913) | |
| Open field | 26.7 (257) | 18.6 (914) | |
| Type of housing | | | |
| Thatched hut | 2.1(20) | 1.2 (61) | |
| Masonry Building | 67.2 (646) | 63.4 (3,115) | 0.007 |
| Block of flats | 26.8 (258) | 29.9 (1,469) | |
| Bungalow | 3.9 (37) | 5.4 (265) | |
| Per capita annual income (in ₹.) | | | |
| ≤300 | 11.1 (96) | 7.8 (339) | |
| 301–500 | 19.2 (165) | 15.0 (652) | |
| 501–800 | 26.9 (232) | 23.6 (1,024) | <0.001 |
| 801–1000 | 12.8 (110) | 13.0 (565) | |
| 1001–1500 | 16.3 (140) | 18.2 (790) | |
| >1500 | 13.7 (118) | 22.3 (965) | |
| Maternal education | | | |
| Illiterate | 41.5 (371) | 30.1 (1,378) | |
| Primary | 17.3 (155) | 16.2 (740) | |
| Middle | 16.4 (147) | 16.0 (732) | <0.001 |
| Matric | 13.5 (121) | 23.3 (1,065) | |
| College | 11.2 (100) | 14.5 (664) | |
| Maternal age at childbirth (years) | | | |
| ≤19 | 8.1 (69) | 8.1 (347) | |
| 20–24 | 36.6 (310) | 35.0 (1,501) | |

(Table 2.2.2 *continued*)

(Table 2.2.2 *continued*)

| | Gestation (weeks) | | |
|---|---|---|---|
| | Preterm Gestation <37 weeks | Term Preterm Gestation ≥37–41 weeks | |
| | % (n) | % (n) | P value |
| 25–29 | 29.6 (251) | 33.6 (1,441) | 0.094 |
| 30–34 | 16.3 (138) | 16.1 (689) | |
| 35+ | 9.3 (79) | 7.3 (311) | |
| Maternal age at marriage (years) | | | |
| <16 | 38.8(287) | 32.1 (1,232) | |
| 16–19 | 31.6 (234) | 32.6 (1,251) | |
| 20–25 | 28.2 (209) | 32.8 (1,259) | <0.001 |
| >25 | 1.4 (10) | 2.6 (100) | |
| Antenatal care | | | |
| Yes | 22.5 (225) | 29.5 (1,485) | |
| No | 77.5 (777) | 70.5 (3,552) | <0.001 |
| Place of delivery | | | |
| Safdarjung Hospital | 25.8 (296) | 23.9 (1,412) | |
| Home | 37.4 (430) | 31.0 (1,830) | |
| Other hospital | 28.5 (327) | 34.9 (2,061) | <0.001 |
| MCH centre | 0.7 (8) | 1.4 (84) | |
| Nursing home | 2.1 (24) | 3.0 (175) | |
| Others | 5.6 (64) | 5.9 (349) | |
| Type of delivery | | | |
| Normal | 93.8 (1,032) | 92.9 (5,386) | |
| Breech | 2.0 (22) | 1.2 (68) | |
| Forceps on vertex | 2.0 (22) | 3.1 (179) | 0.028 |
| C-section | 1.6 (18) | 2.4 (137) | |
| Others | 0.5 (6) | 0.5 (29) | |
| Parity | | | |
| Primipara | 19.6 (140) | 18.7 (701) | |
| Multipara | 80.4 (576) | 81.3 (3,050) | 0.602 |

*Source:* Author.

**Figure 2.2.3:**
*Factors influencing gestation*

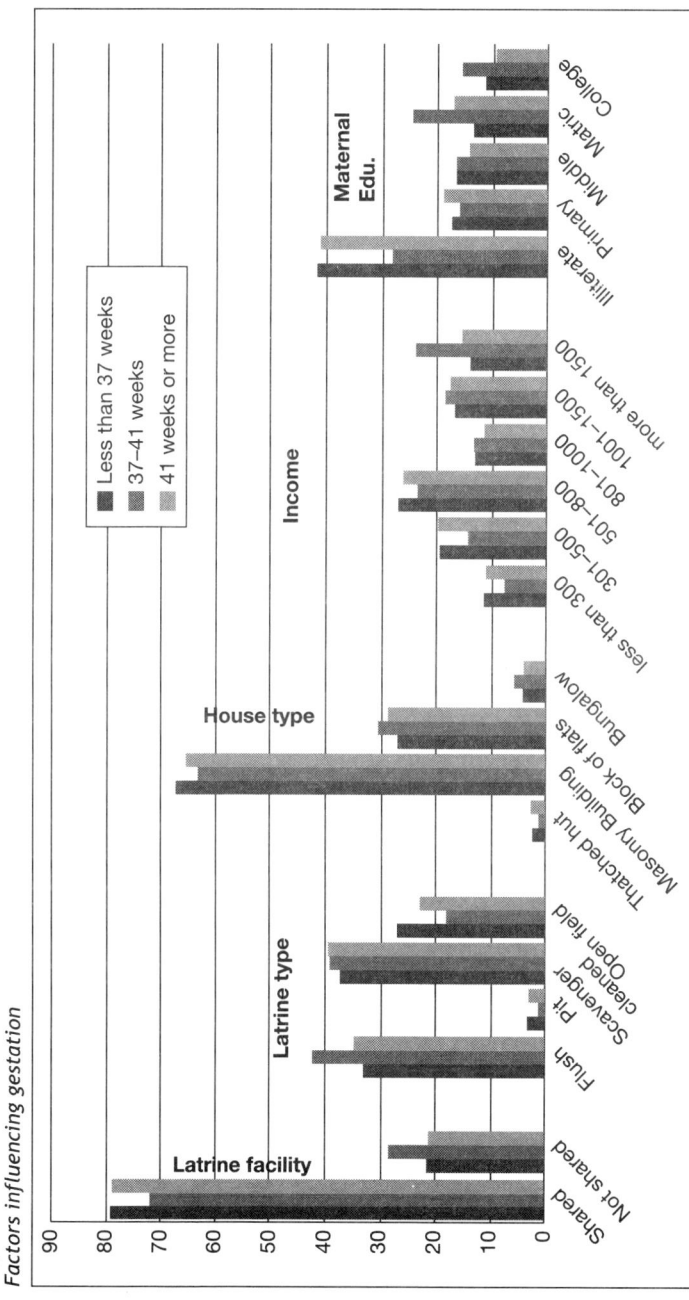

## Size at Birth

Amongst the 8,181 births which were enrolled for this study, birth measurements were recorded in 6,838 (83.5%). The mean birth weight was 2,790 g, length 48.3 cm (centimetres) and head circumference 33.5 cm. The males had significantly higher measurements for all the three parameters (Table 2.2.3).

## Birth Weight

Birth weight of a newly born infant has always remained of tremendous interest and concern to parents and their families. For centuries, it has been a subject of research, public health interest, and debate. This is because birth weight is easy to measure and its ready availability makes it an indicator of population and national health. It is now generally accepted as a reliable indicator of immediate and late outcome of survival and later the well-being of an infant.

Birth weight has been used for a long time for categorization of newborns into normal or high risk. The normal infants have birth weight of 2,500 g or more and the high risk with a birth weight less than 2500g. The WHO, in 1961, defined the infants with birth weight of less than 2,500 g as LBW.

Table 2.2.3:
*Birth measurements mean weight, length, and head circumference in both sexes in cohort subjects*

|  | Total | | Male | | Female | | |
|---|---|---|---|---|---|---|---|
|  | N | *Mean (SD)* | N | *Mean (SD)* | N | *Mean (SD)* | *P Value\** |
| Birth weight (g) | 6838 | 2,790.6 (447.2) | 3603 | 2,827.2 (457.5) | 3235 | 2,749.9 (431.9) | < **0.001** |
| Birth length (cm) | 6645 | 48.3 (2.2) | 3449 | 48.5 (2.3) | 3196 | 48.0 (2.2) | < **0.001** |
| Head circumference (cm) | 6117 | 33.5 (1.3) | 3195 | 33.7 (1.3) | 2922 | 33.3 (1.2) | < **0.001** |

**Source:** Author.

**Note:** * P value for gender difference.

## Birth Measurements

### *Birth Weight*

In the NDBC, the birth measurements were obtained within 72 hours of birth. The mean birth weight for male infant was 2,827.2 g and for female infant 2,749.9 g. The NDBC birth weights were slightly higher than those reported in hospital births and rural studies. However, the mean birth weight of the NDBC cohort is comparable to a recent rigidly controlled, urban, cohort, hospital-based study from Nagpur in which the mean birth weight was 2.9 kg [32,33]. This is an interesting observation as the NDBC study was done almost 40 years ago and it seems the mean birth weight of Indian children remains almost the same and is unchanged.

The maximum number of births (43.3%) occurred in the birth weight group of 2,500–3,000 g. The prevalence of infants with birth weight of 2,500 g or less or LBW was 26.2%. Very few infants were born with birth weight of 4,000 kg or more.

## Length

The mean length of the cohort infants was 48.3 cm with males measuring 48.8 cm and female 48.2 cm. The babies in the Nagpur study have a mean length of 48.6 cm ± 1.8 cm and are slightly taller. About 10% or 8.4% of the babies in the cohort had length shorter than 46 cm and tall babies with length of 53 cm or more were only 1.7%. The proportion of short length infants is comparable to other studies from India and the developing world.

### *Head Circumference*

The mean head circumference of the babies at birth was 33.63 cm. Male and females measured 33.84 and 33.41 cm respectively. In 2.6%, the head size was 32 cm or less and in 8.0% a head size larger than 35.0 cm (Table 2.2.3). In the Nagpur study, infants had slightly a smaller head size with a mean of 33.1 cm [32, 33].

## Factors Influencing Size at Birth

Amongst the three main parameters of body size, namely, weight, height, and head circumference, birth weight seemed to be the most influenced by the environment, socio-economic and educational status of the family, and maternal biological factors such as age, height, pregravid weight, and nutrition. Pregnancy factors such as parity, birth interval of 2 years or less between two successive pregnancies, and pregnancy complications such as anaemia also adversely influenced the body size. The ideal Indian mother should be 20 years or more in age but not elderly, have a weight of more than 45 kg, height greater than 145 cm, birth interval of two or more years between two successive pregnancies, parity varying between 2 and 5, and maternal haemoglobin of greater than 11 g/dl (gram per decilitre).

## Intrauterine Growth

Foetal growth measurement is now recognized as an important parameter to assess the progress on the development of the foetus in uterus. It has been shown to help identify, anticipate, and predict immediate and late outcomes in lives after birth. It is now measured by ultrasound, but in earlier years it was recorded by measuring the height of the uterus from symphysis pubis of the pelvic bone or by measuring the girth of the abdomen. These were useful but were crude and unreliable methods of assessments. In the 1960s, Lubchenco and his colleagues reported for the first time intrauterine growth by measuring the weight, height, and head circumference of the newborns after birth, plotting them with gestational age, and constructing what is now known as intrauterine growth curves. These curves provided clues as to whether the baby had slow, retarded, or fast and accelerated intrauterine growth. In 1971, Ghosh and Bhargava et al. [31] published the first Indian intrauterine growth curves from Safdarjung Hospital, New Delhi. The NDBC, which is an urban cohort with prospectively collected data from pre-pregnant state, also collected similar information. The NDBC intrauterine curves for weight, height, and head circumference are shown in Table 2.2.4 and Figures 2.2.4, 2.2.5, and 2.2.6. These curves provided an opportunity to compare the foetal growth of Indian infants with those from other parts of the country, different socio-economic groups and regions, and at international

**Table 2.2.4:**
*Mean birth weight, length, and head circumference at different gestation period in cohort subjects*

| Gestation (weeks) | Birth Weight (g) | | Birth Length (cm) | | Head Circumference (cm) | |
|---|---|---|---|---|---|---|
| | *N* | *Mean* | *N* | *Mean* | *N* | *Mean* |
| 31 (<=31) | 63 | 2,600.5 (605.5) | 58 | 47.2 (3.2) | 45 | 33.2 (1.8) |
| 34 (32–34) | 280 | 2,618.0 (565.0) | 267 | 47.6 (2.6) | 196 | 33.1 (1.5) |
| 36 (35–36) | 515 | 2,640.3 (465.5) | 503 | 47.5 (2.5) | 452 | 33.1 (1.3) |
| 37 | 475 | 2,666.0 (414.1) | 465 | 47.6 (2.2) | 420 | 33.1 (1.3) |
| 38 | 860 | 2,734.0 (401.0) | 834 | 48.1 (2.1) | 771 | 33.4 (1.2) |
| 39 | 1,208 | 2,812.7 (396.8) | 1,168 | 48.3 (2.0) | 1,113 | 33.5 (1.2) |
| 40 | 1,187 | 2,899.3 (425.1) | 1,161 | 48.7 (2.1) | 1,095 | 33.8 (1.2) |
| 41 | 712 | 2,882.6 (429.7) | 696 | 48.7 (2.1) | 655 | 33.8 (1.2) |
| 42 | 339 | 2,883.0 (462.8) | 332 | 48.7 (2.1) | 315 | 33.7 (1.2) |
| 43 | 195 | 2,854.4 (447.2) | 189 | 48.6 (2.4) | 176 | 33.7 (1.3) |
| 44 | 137 | 2,853.9 (417.8) | 133 | 48.5 (2.0) | 130 | 33.7 (1.2) |
| 45 | 80 | 2,905.4 (427.5) | 76 | 48.8 (2.0) | 70 | 33.7 (1.2) |
| Total | 6,051 | 2,796.8 (442.7) | 5,882 | 48.3 (2.2) | 5,438 | 33.5 (1.2) |

*Source:* Author.

level with other countries. It was interesting to see that the foetal growth of the Ghosh and Bhargava and NDBC infants compared well until 34 weeks of pregnancy with those from western countries. But, thereafter, the foetal growth of the Indian infants slowed and the curves begins to flatten out. It suggested that something happens around 34 weeks of the pregnancy which interferes or interrupts the foetal growth, resulting in smaller Indian infants at birth. It is possible the Indian population had larger number of preterm infants or as pointed out have factors which influence or cause foetal growth retardation. The NDBC growth curves also followed a similar pattern.

In 2009, the WHO constituted the INTERGROWTH-21st group to develop multi-country, population-based intrauterine growth curves for international reference which could be universally used by all countries. This followed the successful development of WHO multicountry growth reference standards (MGRS) in which six countries including India participated, with rigid control on the enrolment of children for the study. The MGRS are international growth standards for children

**Figure 2.2.4:**
*Percentile intrauterine growth curve for weight of the cohort subjects*

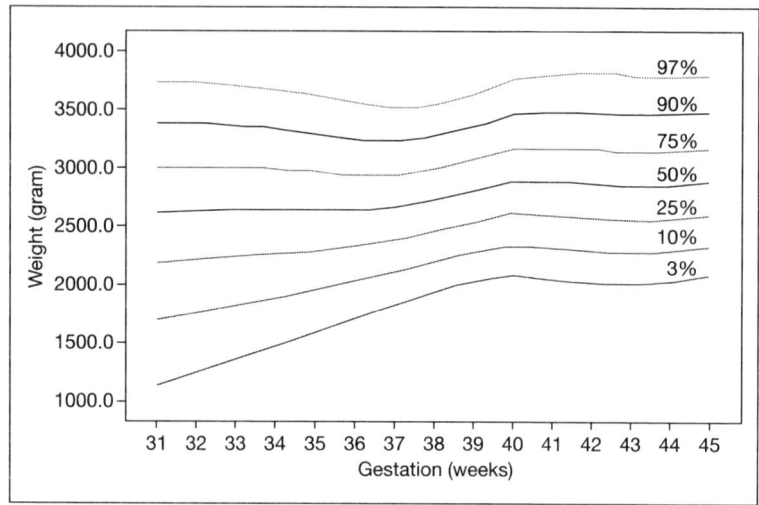

*Source:* Author.

**Figure 2.2.5:**
*Percentile intrauterine growth curve for length of the cohort subjects*

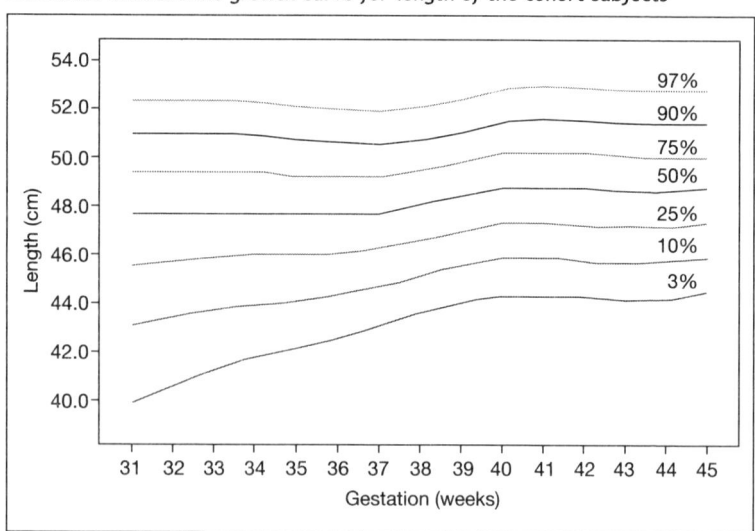

*Source:* Author.

**Figure 2.2.6:**
*Percentile intrauterine growth curve for head circumference of the cohort subjects*

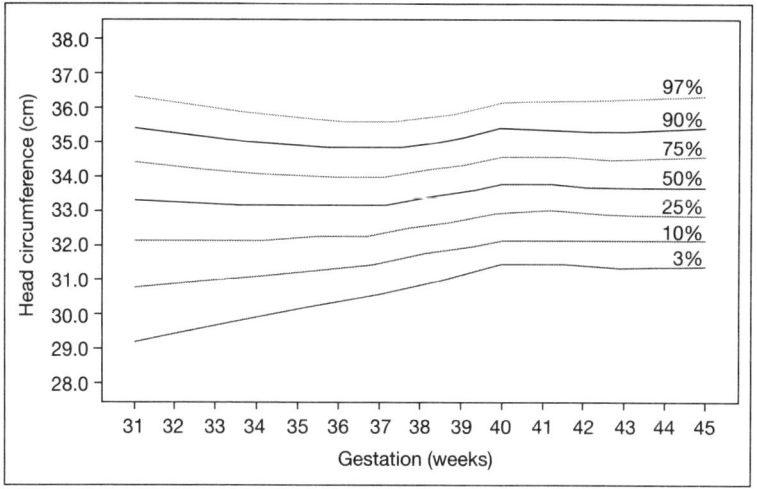

*Source:* Author.

younger than 5 years and which are now accepted and used world over as standard of growth.

INTERGROWTH-21st had eight countries including a centre from Nagpur in India which participated in the study [32]. These collected the data by rigid geographical, clinical, pregnancy, and other parameters and recruited pregnant women who were at minimal or no risk of causing impaired foetal growth. The group published the Newborn Cross-Sectional Study of the 'INTERGROWTH-21st international standards for newborn weight, length, and head circumference by gestational age and sex: The newborn cross-sectional study of the inter growth' [33]. These are currently referred and recommended for use as standards for intrauterine growth of foetus and newborn.

The intrauterine growth is now usually measured by foetal ultra-sonography in pregnancy follow-up, and the paediatrician and newborn specialists (neonatologists) use intrauterine growth from their region or institution and or use WHO INTERGROWTH-21st as reference.

A comparison of INTERGROWTH-21st and NDBC and Ghosh and Bhargava et al. Safdarjung hospital-based growth curves [31] reveal a significant difference beginning from 34 weeks and increasing till 42 weeks of gestation, and the difference is not surprising. The two

**Figure 2.2.7:**

*Comparison of foetal growth curves for birth weight and gestational age of NDBC, Safdarjung Hospital, and INTERGROWTH-21*

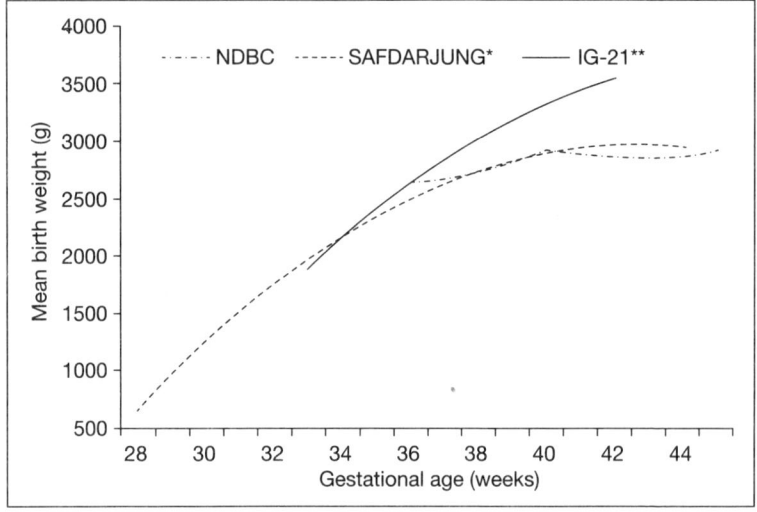

*Source:* Author.
*Note:* *Safdarjung Hospital; ** INTERGROWTH-21.

growth curves have been constructed almost three decades later with striking transitional changes in nutrition, wellness, and environment. (Figure 2.2.7).

# 3

# Low Birth Weight

## Introduction

Low Birth Weight (LBW) is a major public health problem nationally and internationally. It is believed that almost 30% of newborns or every third infant born in India is of LBW. Globally, it is believed that almost 2 million babies are born LBW and almost 300,000 die annually. For a long time, low weight has been considered a risk to survival. But from the 1950s and the 1960s, as interest in this problem grew, it became evident that the LBW caused or contributed to the occurrence of conditions which not only endangered lives but also affected the quality of lives amongst survivors. The suspected LBW infants are at risk from conception to adult life. If the pregnancy is at risk of a LBW infant, it necessitates special attention during pregnancy for both the mother and the unborn including specialised antenatal care and treatment of pregnancy complications, which may need a specialist team of doctors during delivery and at the birth of the newborn. At birth, this newborn may need special assistance for breathing and later neonatal intensive or specialized newborn care depending on whether the baby is preterm or severely growth retarded. During neonatal intensive care, the infant is at perpetual risk to complications, and after survival may have sequelae in terms of brain or lung damage, physical disabilities, poor cognitive function with or without language, and visual and other motor and sensory deficits. The child may need special education because of learning disabilities and may also need more medical consultations, visits, and hospitalizations as compared to its peers. In adult life, the child is at risk of developing chronic disease such as diabetes, coronary artery disease (CAD), blood pressure, and other diseases. LBW is also a known risk for poor human capital development. The total cost for a LBW infant over a life cycle to a family and to the government is many times more than that of the normal child. Furthermore, the family and the mother may go through psycho-social problems include stress, anxiety, and depression.

## Historical Perspective of Low Birth Weight

The term LBW and premature were used interchangeably between the 1920s and the 1950s. In 1961, the WHO defined these as infants who are born with a birth weight of less than 2,500 g irrespective of their period of gestation [34]. Earlier, the terms used were immature and premature and it was believed that all these babies are born early. However, in the 1950s, it was realised that LBW are not homogeneous groups but comprise those born earlier than 37 weeks and those born after 37 weeks or more of gestation but had LBW. In the 1960s, Lubchenco and her colleagues published their work on intrauterine growth curves using birth weight and gestation [35]. The same was published on North Indian babies by Ghosh and Bhargava et al. from India in 1971 [31]. This lead many to suggest classification of infants into those with birth weight appropriate for gestation age (AGA) if the birth weight was in the range of 10–90th centile of expected gestation; Intrauterine growth retarded or small for gestation age (SGA) or intrauterine growth retardation (IUGR) if the birth weight was less than 10th centile for their gestation and large for gestation (LGA) if the birth weight was above 90th centile for gestation [24]. Thus, infants at birth became preterm, term, and post-term AGA, SGA, or LGA.

The NDBC study was primarily planned to prospectively study the problem of LBW which was then and still remains a major public health concern at national and international levels. It is more so in South Asian countries including India and some other developing countries of the world. It is simply because it happens to be the most important underlying or direct cause of childhood morbidity and mortality. This study was expected to provide information on prevalence of low birth, its composition of preterm and SGA infants, and factors contributing to its causation from a representative urban community representing different strata of the society in income, education, and environment and living conditions. The NDBC emanated from a population of 119,799 with 23,700 families residing in a 12 sq km area of South Delhi representing all strata of society, environmental conditions, and health care facilities.

In India, Dr Shanti Ghosh, one of the founders of the NDBC was amongst the first few paediatricians to raise a concern regarding the WHO definition of LBW. She pointed out that these babies are not a homogenous group but comprise infants who are born early or preterm with gestation less than 37 weeks and a significant number of full term infants with gestation 37 weeks or more with intrauterine growth retardation who needed to be supervised care but not total care in special neonatal nurseries. She strongly advocated 2,000 g or less than a cut off for LBW care in newborn care nurseries. [21].

## Prevalence

The prevalence of LBW varies widely across the globe between developed and developing countries, within developing countries, and within the different parts of the same country. It also varies a great deal between urban, rural, or urban poor and urban slum population. In India, it varies from 10–56% in different parts of the country and community [36]. The prevalence also varies depending on the use of cut-off weight for defining LBW for the study, as some have used 2,000 g or less than cut off and others used the international definition of LBW. In India too, this variation and debate had continued for many decades. In the NDBC, the international definition of LBW (birth weight <2,500 g) has been used.

The NDBC recorded high (26.2%) LBW (birth weight <2500 g) prevalence. When the LBW group was further divided into sub-groups, it was noted that infants with birth weight 1,500 g or less were only 0.6 %, those between 1,501 and 2,000 g were 3.4%, and those between 2,001 and 2,500 g were 22.2% (Figure 2.3.1). The results are not comparable to the Western countries where the prevalence of LBW is about 10%. It is also at variance with many other reports from India. This may be due to the nature of sample of the subjects in this study as other cohorts belonged to relatively better environment, parental education and income, pregnancy care, and other factors.

**Figure 2.3.1:**
*Distribution in different birth weight groups*

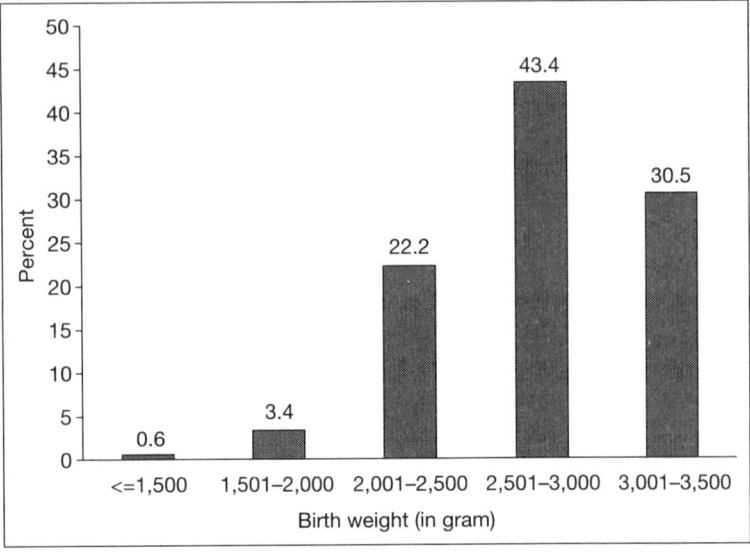

*Source:* Author.

## Birth Weight and Gestation

The LBW comprised both preterm and term infants. In all the birth weight groups we found preterm and term infants, and there was a distinct overlap between these two groups of infants. In the birth weight group of 1,500 g or less, 66.7% were preterm and 32.3% were term or post-term. In the next higher birth weight group of 1,501–2,000 g, the preterm were 40.6% and term or post-term were 60.4%. In the group 2,001–2,500 g, the preterm were only 18.5% and remaining were term or post-term. Thereafter, in larger groups too, preterm were seen but these were fewer. Overall, the preterm contributed to about 15% and over 85% or more were term growth retarded or SGA age (term SGA). Most of the preterm were from late preterm gestation group of 34 weeks to 36 weeks of gestation (Figure 2.3.2).

## Intrauterine Growth

The foetal growth measurements were available in 6,051 infants. Amongst these, the prevalence of infants with birth weight AGA was

**Figure 2.3.2:**
*Distribution by birth weight and gestational age*

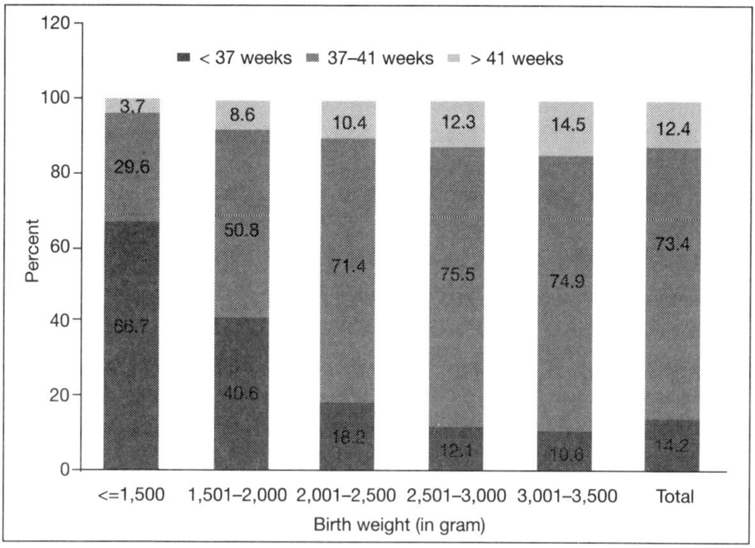

*Source:* Author.

81.2%, SGA was 9.4%, and LGA was 9.2%. The length was AGA in 82.5%, short or stunted in 8.9%, and LGA in 8.5%.

## Causative Factors of Low Birth Weight

LBW is known to be caused by multiple factors varying from genetic to environment, family, socio-cultural, economic and educational status, maternal health from pre-pregnant state to pregnancy, placental causes, and foetal diseases and malformations. These are also caused by infections and newborn morbidities and problems. The NDBC had a high prevalence of LBW in a population selected from all strata of urban life and background. Thus, we found its association with environmental factors such as sanitation, water supply and housing, family education income, socio-cultural patterns such age at marriage, number of children, and interval between two successive pregnancies and maternal biological factors such as age and parity, maternal pregravid nutrition reflected as weight, height and anaemia, and so forth. Table 2.3.1 summarizes the analysis of causes contributing to LBW in the NDBC. It reconfirmed that

**Table 2.3.1:**
*Causes of LBW in cohort subjects*

| Sex | Birth Weight Group (g) | |
|---|---|---|
| | *<2,500 g* | *≥2,500 g* |
| Male | 619 | 2,462 |
| Female | 764 | 2,181 |
| Total | 1,383 | 4,643 |

***P value <0.001***

| Mother's Education | Birth Weight Group (g) | |
|---|---|---|
| Illiterate | 531 | 1,405 |
| Undermatric | 468 | 1,475 |
| Matricultate and above | 384 | 1,743 |
| Total | 1,383 | 4,623 |

***P value <0.001***

| Age of the Mother | Birth Weight Group (g) | |
|---|---|---|
| <20 | 28 | 156 |
| 20–34 | 126 | 1,704 |
| 35–39 | 8 | 62 |
| 40+ | 3 | 14 |
| Total | 165 | 1,936 |

***P value 0.0002***

| Mother's Height (cm) | Birth Weight Group (g) | |
|---|---|---|
| <145 | 127 | 220 |
| 145–149 | 264 | 770 |
| 150–159 | 396 | 1,644 |
| 160 + | 30 | 174 |
| Total | 817 | 2,808 |

***P value <0.001***

| Maternal Parity | Birth Weight Group (g) | |
|---|---|---|
| 1 | 382 | 912 |
| 2–4 | 720 | 2,746 |
| 5+ | 281 | 985 |
| Total | 1,383 | 4,643 |

***P value <0.001***

| Haemoglobin Level (g) | Birth Weight Group (g) | |
|---|---|---|
| <8 | 15 | 86 |
| 8–10 | 27 | 236 |
| 10 | 9 | 98 |
| Total | 51 | 420 |
| **P value 0.297** | | |

**Source:** Author.

the birth weight is influenced by environment, socio-economics, maternal education and nutrition, maternal health before and during pregnancy, pregnancy complications, and foetal malformations.

The distinctive feature about these causes is that most of them are preventable by simple practical and low-cost interventions. Amongst the most important preventable causes and possible intervention include the age at marriage and first pregnancy to be beyond 20 years; birth interval between two successive pregnancies to be more than 2 years; diagnosis, treatment, and prevention of maternal anaemia; improving antenatal care attendance in all trimesters with early registration of pregnancy at a health care facility; and to ensure that the mother had received education until at least primary or middle school. An expectant mother should be made to rest during the day, controlling and treating pregnancy complications such as hypertension, and ensuring potable drinking water with proper sanitation and general housing conditions.

## Outcome of Low Birth Weight

### Mortality

1. **Birth weight**

   The neonatal mortality was generally high in all LBW groups and was inversely related to birth weight. It was noted that lower the birth weight the higher was the mortality. In the LBW group (2,500 g or less) the mortality was 13.2 times (95% CI 2.3, 4.5 $p < 0.001$) higher as compared to normal birth weight infants. Stratification in birth weight groups of 500g each, it was 100% in the infants with birth weight 1,000 g or less and decreased sharply to less than half to 46.1% in birth weight group of 1,001–1,500 g or less. It further showed a decline by 1/3rd to 15.04% in the birth weight group of 1,501–2,000 g and to a mere 2.2% in birth weight group of 2,001–2,500 g. (Figure 2.3.3). However, even in this group infants are known to die 4–10 times more often than infants with birth weight more than 2,500 g. It was interesting to note that for the same birth weight the mortality was low if the gestational age was higher. Thus in birth weight groups 1,501–2,000 g the mortality for preterm was 21.4% as compared to 14.2% for term infants. A similar trend was visible in the birth weight group of 2,001–2,500 g where the preterm mortality was 3 times higher. When compared to the Safdarjung hospital from New Delhi and other parts of the country, the mortality in the NDBC was significantly lower except for the very LBW group.

2. **Gestation**

The overall mortality for the preterm was high. It is high as compared to that reported in the Indian literature [5, 6, 8, 11, 12] as 25.0% in 1,000–1,500 g, 13.5% in 1,501–1,999 g, and 3.0% in 2,000–2,499 g. The relationship between gestation and mortality was similar to the birth weight. It was inversely related to gestational age; the lower the gestation higher the mortality (Figure 2.3.4). However, for the same birth weight, shorter gestation babies had a significantly higher mortality.

**Figure 2.3.3:**
*Neonatal mortality rate per 1,000 births in different birth weight groups*

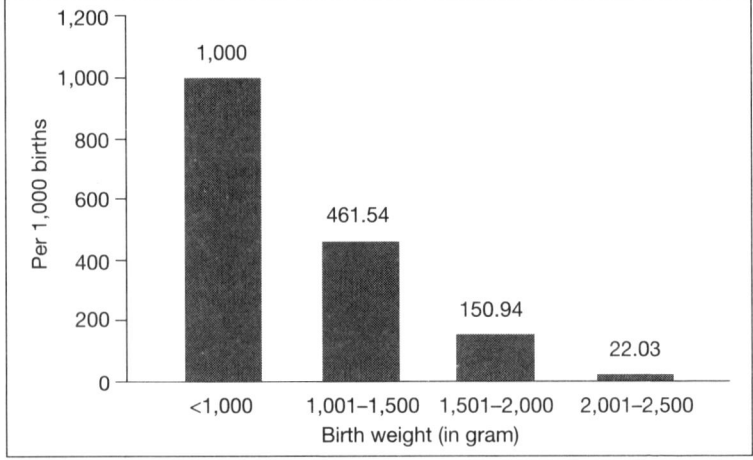

*Source:* Author.

3. **By Intrauterine Growth**

   IUGR seemed to influence the mortality significantly. Neonatal mortality was high in IUGR or SGA infants as compared to AGA and LGA infants. This was almost five times the AGA group and 10 times the LGA group. The same pattern was continued in infancy and in under five and later (P < 0.001; Table 2.3.2).

## Causes of Morbidity and Mortality

This was a field study and, therefore, it was not possible to record the immediate or late causes of morbidity and mortality. The information that was gathered was from discharged hospital records or as reported by recollections by the parents. The commonly reported causes of death were prematurity, asphyxia, respiratory distress, infections, and malformations. These are consistent with those described in the literature.

**Figure 2.3.4:**
*Neonatal mortality rate per 1,000 births in different birth weight groups by gestation*

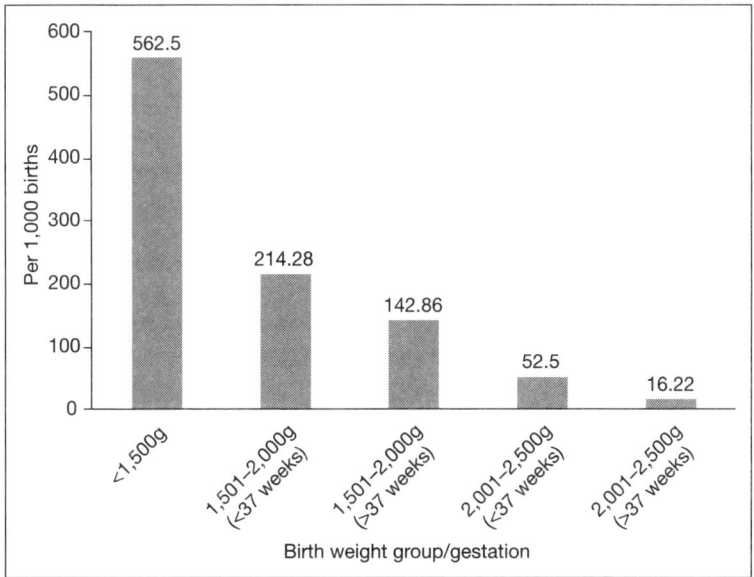

*Source:* Author.

**Table 2.3.2:**
*Mortality pattern and intrauterine growth in cohort subjects*

| | Weight | |
|---|---|---|
| *Intrauterine Growth Group* | *Number* | *Death* (%)* |
| SGA (<10th centile) | 574 | 13.6 |
| AGA (10–90th centile) | 4,915 | 2.8 |
| LGA (>90th centile) | 562 | 1.6 |

**Source:** Author.
**Note:** * P value < 0.001

However, the literature also describes specific causes which are more prevalent in preterm and SGA age infants. Those which are common in shorter gestation or preterm are hyaline membrane disease and brain haemorrhage and those with SGA are lung haemorrhage and congenital malformations. Birth asphyxia and infections are common to all LBW irrespective of IUGR or gestational age. Fever, diarrhoeas, pneumonia, skin infections, and ear infectious were the commonly reported causes of morbidity in later childhood.

## Physical Growth

The physical growth of the LBW infant which included both preterm and intrauterine growth retarded was significantly lower in both boys and girls, as compared to non-LBW peers. These LBW were born with significantly lower birth weight, length, and head circumference and remained significantly smaller throughout childhood to attainment of adulthood (Tables 2.3.3 and 2.3.4) and showed no evidence of catch up growth at any age period.

Even amongst the different LBW groups of <2,000 g, 2,000–2,499 g, and >2,500 g the mean weight, height, and head circumference at different age periods from birth to adulthood showed highly significant differences (Tables 2.3.5 and 2.3.6, $p < 0.001$). None of the LBW groups showed a catch up or faster growth [5, 8] (Figures 2.3.5, 2.3.6, and 2.3.7).

These observations are consistent with other studies reported in the literature. The most distinctive and striking feature about the NDBC

**Table 2.3.3:**
*Mean length/height (cm) comparison in birth weight <2,500 g (LBW) and birth weight ≥2,500 g (normal) in cohort subjects from birth to 20 years at different age periods*

| Age in Years | <2,500 g N | <2,500 g Mean (SD) | ≥2,500 g N | ≥2,500 g Mean (SD) | P Value |
|---|---|---|---|---|---|
| 0 | 1,718 | 46.2 (1.97) | 4,925 | 49.0 (1.9) | <0.001 |
| 0.5 | 1,584 | 62.8 (2.7) | 4,683 | 65.1 (2.5) | <0.001 |
| 1 | 1,175 | 69.5 (3.1) | 3,639 | 71.7 (3.0) | <0.001 |
| 2 | 1,165 | 78.6 (3.7) | 3,698 | 81.1 (3.8) | <0.001 |
| 3 | 1,117 | 86.1 (4.3) | 3,549 | 88.7 (4.3) | <0.001 |
| 4 | 1,055 | 93.1 (4.5) | 3,366 | 95.6 (4.4) | <0.001 |
| 5 | 919 | 99.7 (4.6) | 3,023 | 102.1 (4.7) | <0.001 |
| 11 | 684 | 133.7 (6.7) | 2,332 | 136.1 (6.7) | <0.001 |
| 15 | 659 | 154.9 (8.0) | 2,197 | 157.9 (8.0) | <0.001 |
| 20 | 189 | 160.1 (9.1) | 654 | 164.0 (8.8) | <0.001 |

*Source:* Author.

**Table 2.3.4:**
*Mean weight (kg) comparison in birth weight <2,500 g (LBW) and birth weight ≥2,500 g (normal) in cohort subjects from birth to 20 years at different age periods*

| Age in Years | <2,500 g N | <2,500 g Mean (SD) | ≥2,500 g N | ≥2,500 g Mean (SD) | P Value |
|---|---|---|---|---|---|
| 0 | 1,783 | 2.25 (0.25) | 5,055 | 2.98 (0.33) | <0.001 |
| 0.5 | 1,590 | 6.02 (0.90) | 4,688 | 6.91 (0.89) | <0.001 |
| 1 | 1,176 | 7.55 (1.06) | 3,643 | 8.42 (1.14) | <0.001 |
| 2 | 1,165 | 9.39 (1.18) | 3,669 | 10.34 (1.35) | <0.001 |
| 3 | 1,110 | 11.21 (1.42) | 3,524 | 12.20 (1.50) | <0.001 |
| 4 | 1,049 | 12.95 (1.62) | 3,351 | 14.0 (1.64) | <0.001 |
| 5 | 921 | 14.46 (1.72) | 3,028 | 15.52 (1.83) | <0.001 |
| 11 | 685 | 26.77 (4.92) | 2,337 | 28.88 (5.29) | <0.001 |
| 15 | 660 | 43.14 (7.92) | 2,202 | 46.35 (8.71) | <0.001 |
| 20 | 189 | 160.08 (9.07) | 654 | 163.95 (8.83) | <0.001 |

*Source:* Author.

**Table 2.3.5:**

*Mean weight (kg) for different categories of birth weight in cohort subjects at different age periods*

| Age in Years | *<2,000 g* N | Mean (SD) | *2,000–2,499 g* N | Mean (SD) | *≥2,500 g* N | Mean (SD) | P Value |
|---|---|---|---|---|---|---|---|
| 0 | 268 | 1.77 (0.23) | 1,515 | 2.33 (0.13) | 5,055 | 2.98 (0.33) | <0.001 |
| 0.5 | 196 | 5.34 (0.89) | 1,394 | 6.11 (0.86) | 4,688 | 6.91 (0.89) | <0.001 |
| 1 | 139 | 6.97 (1.12) | 1,037 | 7.63 (1.03) | 3,643 | 8.42 (1.14) | <0.001 |
| 2 | 130 | 8.87 (1.14) | 1,035 | 9.46 (1.17) | 3,669 | 10.34 (1.35) | <0.001 |
| 3 | 125 | 10.6 (1.39) | 985 | 11.29 (1.40) | 3,524 | 12.20 (1.50) | <0.001 |
| 4 | 114 | 12.4 (1.68) | 935 | 13.03 (1.60) | 3,351 | 13.97 (1.64) | <0.001 |
| 5 | 100 | 13.76 (1.76) | 821 | 14.55 (1.70) | 3,028 | 15.52 (1.83) | <0.001 |
| 11 | 69 | 25.72 (4.86) | 616 | 26.89 (4.91) | 2,337 | 28.87 (5.29) | <0.001 |
| 15 | 66 | 41.37 (7.34) | 594 | 43.34 (7.96) | 2,202 | 46.35 (8.71) | <0.001 |
| 20 | 11 | 158.96 (11.14) | 178 | 160.15 (8.96) | 654 | 163.95 (8.83) | <0.001 |

*Source:* Author.

**Table 2.3.6:**

*Mean length/height (cm) for different categories of birth weight in cohort subjects at different age periods*

| Age in Years | *<2,000 g* N | Mean (SD) | *2,000–2,499 g* N | Mean (SD) | *≥2,500 g* N | Mean (SD) | P Value |
|---|---|---|---|---|---|---|---|
| 0 | 239 | 43.9 (2.3) | 1,479 | 46.6 (1.6) | 4,925 | 49.0 (1.9) | <0.001 |
| 0.5 | 193 | 60.4 (2.8) | 1,391 | 63.1 (2.5) | 4,683 | 65.1 (2.5) | <0.001 |
| 1 | 138 | 67.7 (3.2) | 1,037 | 69.7 (3.0) | 3,639 | 71.7 (3.0) | <0.001 |
| 2 | 129 | 76.7 (3.8) | 1,036 | 78.9 (3.6) | 3,698 | 81.1 (3.8) | <0.001 |
| 3 | 125 | 84.2 (4.5) | 992 | 86.4 (4.3) | 3,549 | 88.7 (4.3) | <0.001 |
| 4 | 115 | 91.6 (4.6) | 940 | 93.3 (4.4) | 3,366 | 95.6 (4.4) | <0.001 |
| 5 | 99 | 98.1 (5.1) | 820 | 99.9 (4.5) | 3,023 | 102.1 (4.7) | <0.001 |
| 11 | 69 | 132.5 (7.4) | 615 | 133.8 (6.6) | 2,332 | 136.1 (6.7) | <0.001 |
| 15 | 66 | 153.4 (7.7) | 593 | 155.1 (8.1) | 2,197 | 157.9 (8.0) | <0.001 |
| 20 | 11 | 159.0 (11.1) | 178 | 160.1 (9.0) | 654 | 164.0 (8.8) | <0.001 |

*Source:* Author.

**Figure 2.3.5:**
*Birth weight and body growth in weight from birth to 20 years in boys*

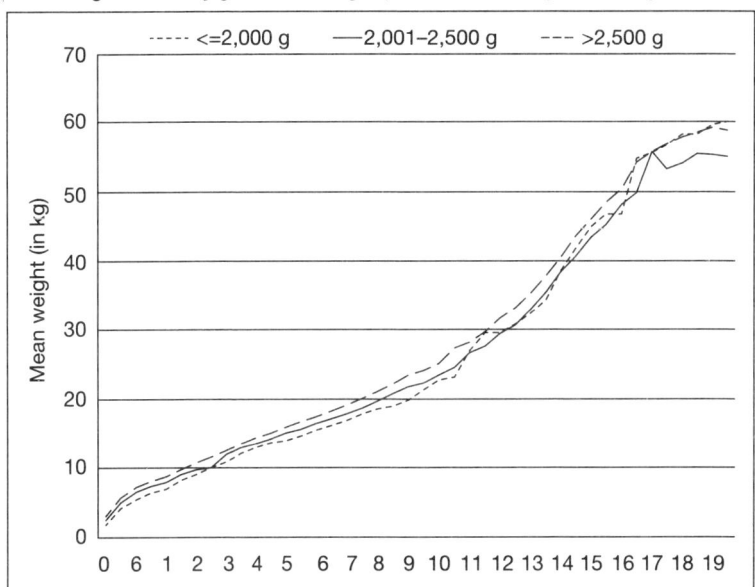

*Source:* Author.

longitudinal studies is that these were several years ahead of their times
and in many ways' were path breaking. Similar observations have been
observed in other studies reported from India and elsewhere [4, 7, 9, 11,
37, 38, 41].

## Gestation and Body Growth

### Preterm

The growth pattern in preterm, when compared to term normal gestation
children, showed an interesting pattern. There was a distinct attempt to
catch up with their peers. The preterm remained smaller in the first
2 years but began to catch up from around 3 years of age. The difference

**Figure 2.3.6:**
*Birth weight and body growth in weight from birth to 20 years in girls*

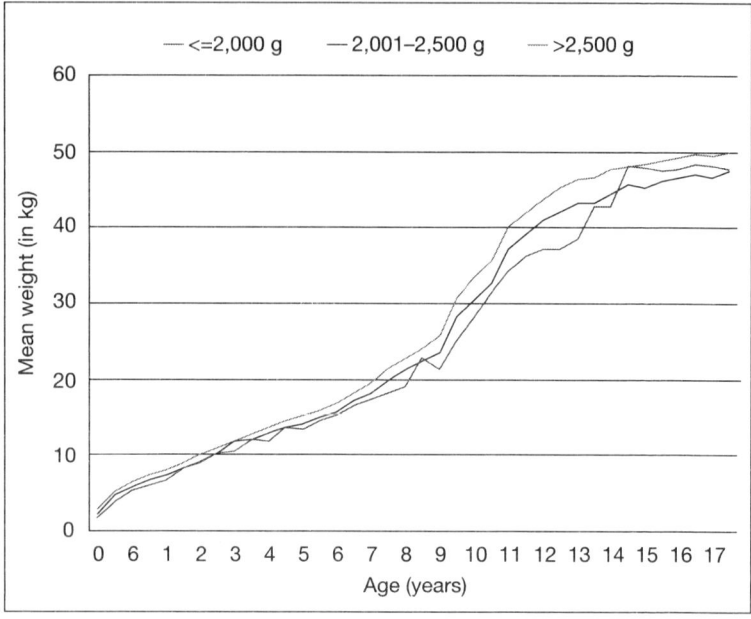

*Source:* Author.

disappearing by 5 years of age, the growth pattern varied at different ages, but by 10 years of age the preterm showed sustained growth and their weight, height, and head circumference was comparable to normal gestation and normal weight children (Table 2.3.7).

It appears that the preterm were able to overcome their disadvantage of an abrupt interruption of growth due to termination of pregnancy. It also seemed logical to assume that whatever be the cause/s which initiated or precipitated the labour, it did not influence the subsequent growth of the preterm provided the preterm otherwise remained normal and did not suffer from any morbidities which could influence body growth. For physical growth, the LBW preterm did not have the same poor outcome as for survival. These observations are consistent with other reports in literature [1, 3, 7, 9, 14, 19, 37, 39, 40, 42].

**Figure 2.3.7:**
*Birth weight and height from birth to 20 years in boys*

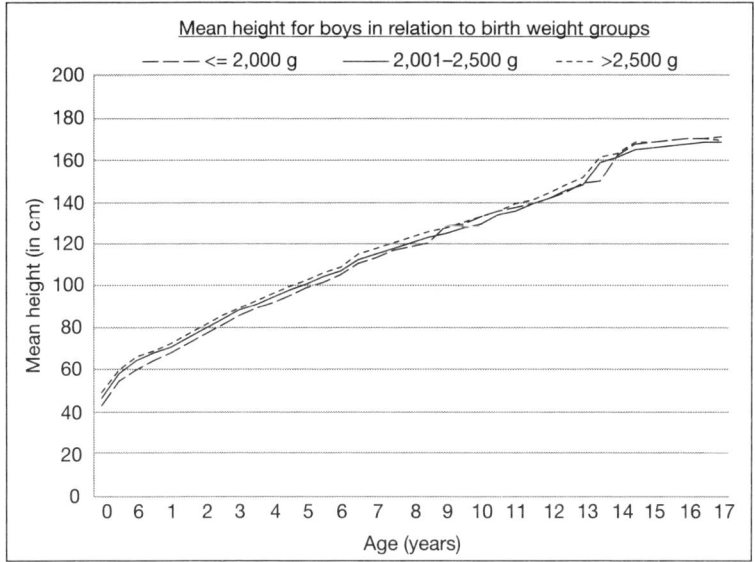

*Source:* Author.

**Table 2.3.7:**
*Preterm and term weight and height growth pattern in cohort subjects*

| | | Gestation (weeks) | | | |
|---|---|---|---|---|---|
| | | <37 | | 37–41 | |
| Age in Years | N | Mean (SD) | N | Mean (SD) | P Value |
| | | Length/Height (cm) | | | |
| 0 | 828 | 47.52 (2.57) | 4,324 | 48.37 (2.13) | <0.001 |
| 0.5 | 874 | 63.87 (2.84) | 4,445 | 64.68 (2.69) | <0.001 |
| 1 | 684 | 70.44 (3.21) | 3,503 | 71.39 (3.15) | <0.001 |
| 2 | 667 | 79.69 (3.92) | 3,519 | 80.84 (3.85) | <0.001 |
| 3 | 647 | 87.29 (4.48) | 3,393 | 88.52 (4.34) | <0.001 |
| 4 | 605 | 94.31 (4.57) | 3,212 | 95.38 (4.49) | <0.001 |
| 5 | 534 | 101.05 (4.78) | 2,865 | 101.89 (4.78) | <0.001 |
| 11 | 399 | 134.70 (6.60) | 2,209 | 135.84 (6.84) | 0.002 |
| 15 | 383 | 156.43 (8.56) | 2,061 | 157.56 (8.11) | 0.002 |
| 20 | 105 | 163.08 (9.11) | 628 | 163.35 (9.03) | 0.146 |

(Table 2.3.7 *continued*)

(Table 2.3.7 *continued*)

| Age in Years | Gestation (weeks) | | | | P Value |
|---|---|---|---|---|---|
| | <37 | | 37–41 | | |
| | N | Mean (SD) | N | Mean (SD) | |
| | | **Weight (kg)** | | | |
| 0 | 858 | 2.63 (0.51) | 4,442 | 2.82 (0.42) | <0.001 |
| 0.5 | 877 | 6.51 (1.02) | 4,450 | 6.75 (0.96) | <0.001 |
| 1 | 683 | 8.00 (1.15) | 3,506 | 8.31 (1.17) | <0.001 |
| 2 | 662 | 9.89 (1.33) | 3,495 | 10.21 (1.37) | <0.001 |
| 3 | 642 | 11.75 (1.54) | 3,375 | 12.07 (1.54) | <0.001 |
| 4 | 600 | 13.53 (1.73) | 3,195 | 13.82 (1.70) | <0.001 |
| 5 | 535 | 15.13 (1.87) | 2,870 | 15.35 (1.89) | 0.004 |
| 11 | 400 | 27.90 (4.97) | 2,211 | 28.60 (5.41) | 0.013 |
| 15 | 383 | 44.75 (8.69) | 2,066 | 45.99 (8.67) | 0.003 |
| 20 | 105 | 53.69 (9.23) | 629 | 54.61 (10.85) | 0.257 |

*Source:* Author.

**Figure 2.3.8:**
*Small for gestation and body growth in body weight from birth to 20 years*

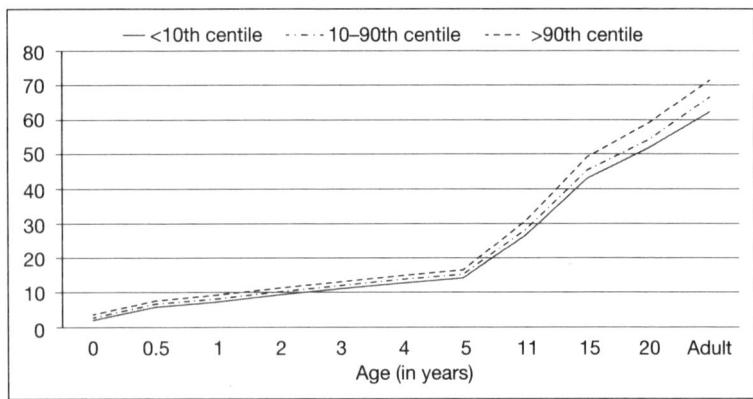

*Source:* Author.

## Small for Gestation and Body Growth

The SGA infants recorded a poor growth pattern as compared to normal and even preterm children (Figure 2.3.8). These infants are born small in size and remain lighter and shorter from childhood to adulthood. There appeared to be some evidence of catch-up growth around 9 years or the pre-pubertal period, but it did not last and finally these children had significantly lower weight and height till full attainment of adulthood. They were almost 4 kg lighter and 3 cm shorter than AGA or normal babies (Tables 2.3.8 and 2.3.9). Later studies have also been consistent with these results [37–44].

**Table 2.3.8:**
*Mean comparison of length/height at different ages among the categories of foetal centiles for length in the cohort subjects*

| Age in | <10th Centile | | 10–90th Centile | | >90th Centile | |
|---|---|---|---|---|---|---|
| Years | N | Mean (SD) | N | Mean (SD) | N | Mean (SD) |
| 0 | 529 | 44.14 (1.53) | 4,853 | 48.34 (1.48) | 500 | 52.18 (1.19) |
| 0.5 | 471 | 61.74 (2.92) | 4,533 | 64.54 (2.44) | 469 | 67.35 (2.18) |
| 1 | 356 | 68.73 (3.12) | 3,513 | 71.12 (2.97) | 373 | 74.08 (2.75) |
| 2 | 368 | 77.81 (3.69) | 3,561 | 80.51 (3.69) | 385 | 83.84 (3.51) |
| 3 | 344 | 85.25 (4.33) | 3,417 | 88.12 (4.23) | 378 | 91.64 (3.85) |
| 4 | 328 | 92.10 (4.45) | 3,245 | 95.01 (4.35) | 354 | 98.41 (4.08) |
| 5 | 286 | 98.56 (4.52) | 2,920 | 101.54 (4.58) | 337 | 104.96 (4.44) |
| 11 | 218 | 131.61 (6.67) | 2,262 | 135.45 (6.58) | 254 | 139.72 (6.29) |
| 15 | 206 | 152.54 (7.75) | 2,129 | 157.04 (7.75) | 241 | 162.45 (8.77) |
| 20 | 67 | 157.78 (8.40) | 625 | 162.84 (8.50) | 62 | 169.68 (8.61) |
| Adult | 100 | 160.05 (9.14) | 1,080 | 163.10 (9.29) | 112 | 168.87 (9.00) |

*Source:* Author.

The comparison of mean at all ages were highly significant with P value <0.001 across the three categories.

**Table 2.3.9:**
*Mean comparison of weight at different ages among the categories of foetal centiles for weight in the cohort subjects*

| Age in | <10th Centile | | 10–90th Centile | | >90th Centile | |
|---|---|---|---|---|---|---|
| Years | N | Mean (SD) | N | Mean (SD) | N | Mean (SD) |
| 0 | 574 | 2.03 (0.25) | 4,915 | 2.80 (0.30) | 562 | 3.59 (0.24) |
| 0.5 | 489 | 5.77 (0.95) | 4,583 | 6.71 (0.89) | 522 | 7.61 (0.88) |
| 1 | 359 | 7.36 (1.10) | 3,559 | 8.22 (1.12) | 425 | 9.18 (1.07) |
| 2 | 364 | 9.20 (1.20) | 3,578 | 10.12 (1.30) | 436 | 11.24 (1.33) |
| 3 | 345 | 10.99 (1.42) | 3,431 | 11.96 (1.48) | 425 | 13.08 (1.44) |

(Table 2.3.9 *continued*)

(Table 2.3.9 *continued*)

| Age in Years | <10th Centile | | 10–90th Centile | | >90th Centile | |
|---|---|---|---|---|---|---|
| | N | Mean (SD) | N | Mean (SD) | N | Mean (SD) |
| 4 | 321 | 12.67 (1.60) | 3,264 | 13.72 (1.63) | 402 | 14.89 (1.54) |
| 5 | 289 | 14.15 (1.71) | 2,943 | 15.25 (1.80) | 367 | 16.56 (1.73) |
| 11 | 216 | 26.55 (5.08) | 2,276 | 28.31 (5.23) | 283 | 30.75 (5.33) |
| 15 | 204 | 43.11 (8.13) | 2,139 | 45.45 (8.54) | 277 | 49.16 (8.72) |
| 20 | 54 | 51.62 (9.25) | 640 | 53.97 (10.52) | 79 | 58.88 (9.70) |
| Adult | 100 | 62.21 (13.71) | 1,089 | 66.53 (15.26) | 117 | 71.46 (13.99) |

*Source:* Author.

The comparison of mean at all ages were highly significant with P value < 0.001 across the three categories.

## Development of Low Birth Weight Children

Developmental assessment of the LBW children was done at several age points. The first was done during 0–2 years, the second at age 4, and the third at 5–6 years of age. In the first 2 years, the children were mainly tested for motor milestones and language development (speech). In general, the motor milestones such as sitting, crawling, standing without support, and walking were achieved in majority by the age of 6 months, crawling between 7 and 8 months, and walking without support by 1 year of age. Almost 60% of the babies began to sit by 6 months, crawl by 7–8 months and walked by 1 year of age. About 5% of the LBW seemed to have delayed sitting by 9–10 months, crawling by 11 months or more, and standing without support by 18 months or more. About 55% of infants were speaking monosyllables by 1 year and about 9% spoke monosyllables after 18–20 months. Birth weight, maternal education, socio-economic status, and body growth seemed to influence early development as children with lower birth weight appeared to achieve the motor milestones such as sitting, crawling, and standing without support later than those with higher birth weight. Interestingly, in various sub-groups of heavier babies, the difference in age at achieving particular milestones was minimal and at times the difference was negligible. For example, whereas the differences between ≤2 kg and 2.1 to <2.5 kg was marked, the difference between 2.1 and 2.5 kg and more than 3 kg was minimal. In general, birth weight, socio-economic, and maternal educational status seemed to influence the development with better performance (Tables 2.3.10 and 2.3.11). Even primary or up to middle level of school education of mother showed significant advancement in achieving milestones as compared to illiterate mothers. Early language development did not appear to be affected by birth weight. However, babies of educated mothers started speaking earlier as compared to babies of non-educated mothers.

The development of the LBW was further tested for the social maturity scale, Central Institute of Education (CIE), verbal test, and CD development test. It showed the mean scores to be within normal limits. However, when compared to controls from similar background but with normal weight, the scores were significantly lower in the LBW infants. It indicated that the LBW infants are at a disadvantage as compared to normal children. The intelligence quotient (IQ) in the LBWs and controls again showed significant differences in favour of the controls (P < 0.001) (Table 2.3.12). Similar findings have been reported by other workers [1, 4, 9, 11, 13, 15, 40, 47].

A distribution of LBW and control children in social quotient or intelligent quotient again revealed interesting findings. Children with LBW in the performance and intelligence tests scored below 90 (subnormal level) in significantly higher numbers. These differences are striking and suggest that the low birth infants to be at distinct disadvantage than normal birth weight children (Tables 2.3.12 and 2.3.13).

The developmental assessment comparison between the preterm and SGA in general did not suggest any significant difference even though the birth weight in the two groups was almost similar. The mean scores in social maturity scales, CIE verbal test, CD performance test, and IQ were within normal range for both the groups, and the differences were not statistically significant. However, when compared to normal infants, the scores in these tests also appeared to be lower in both the groups (Table 2.3.14).

## The Long Term Consequences of Low Birth Weight

### Developmental Origin of Adult Diseases

David Barker in 1994 proposed the hypothesis of 'foetal origin of adult diseases' [17]. It was based on his observations that adults with LBW are prone to early deaths and diseases of the heart such as coronary heart

**Table 2.3.10:**
Intellectual development and mother's socio-economic status in LBW and normal cohort subjects

| S.Q./I.Q. | ₹ 20 Study Group No | % | Control Group No | % | ₹ 21–50 Study Group No | % | Control Group No | % | ₹ 51–100 Study Group No | % | Control Group No | % | ₹ 101–200 Study Group No | % | Control Group No | % | ₹ 101–200 Study Group No | % | Control Group No | % |
|---|---|---|---|---|---|---|---|---|---|---|---|---|---|---|---|---|---|---|---|---|
| ≤90 | – | – | 2 | 2.8 | 16 | 22.2 | 6 | 3.4 | 13 | 18 | 2 | 2.8 | 2 | 3 | 1 | 1 | 1 | 1 | – | – |
| 91–110 | 1 | 1.4 | – | – | – | 6.9 | 13 | 18.3 | 18 | 25 | 22 | 31 | 13 | 18 | 9 | 13 | 2 | 3 | 4 | 6 |
| >110 | – | – | – | – | – | – | 2 | 2.8 | – | – | 6 | 8.4 | 1 | 1 | 3 | 4 | – | – | 1 | 1 |

**Source:** Author.

**Table 2.3.11:**
Intellectual development and mother's educational status in LBW and normal cohort subjects

| S.Q./I.Q. | Illiterate | | | | Primary | | | | High School and Matric | | | | Technical and Graduate | | | |
| | Study Group | | Control | | Study Group | | Control | | Study Group | | Control | | Study Group | | Control | |
| | M | % | M | % | M | % | M | % | M | % | M | % | M | % | M | % |
|---|---|---|---|---|---|---|---|---|---|---|---|---|---|---|---|---|
| ≤90 | 20 | 25 | 4 | 6 | 9 | 11 | 2 | 2.9 | 9 | 11 | 3 | 4.3 | 1 | 1 | – | – |
| 91–110 | 7 | 9 | 13 | 18 | 7 | 9 | 6 | 8.5 | 24 | 30 | 24 | 34.2 | 1 | 1 | 4 | 5.7 |
| >110 | – | – | 1 | 1 | – | – | – | – | 1 | 1.3 | 9 | 12.9 | – | – | 4 | 5.7 |
| Total | 27 | 34 | 18 | 26 | 16 | 20 | 8 | 11 | 34 | 43 | 36 | 51.4 | 2 | 3 | 8 | 11 |

**Source:** Author.

**Table 2.3.12:**
*Mean IQ levels on LBW and normal cohort subjects at 5–6 years of age*

| | | Low Birth Weight | | | | Control | | | Statistical Significance |
|---|---|---|---|---|---|---|---|---|---|
| TESTS | No. | Mean | SD | % | No. | Mean | SD | % | p Value |
| SMS | 149 | 98.3 | 11.7 | – | 117 | 108.06 | 6.24 | – | <0.001 |
| CIE | 159 | 92.9 | 16 | – | 122 | 103.37 | 5.48 | – | <0.001 |
| CD | 58 | 99.3 | 17.8 | – | 46 | 101 | 0.54 | – | >0.05 |

*Source:* Author.

**Table 2.3.13:**
*Intellectual development in LBW and normal cohort subjects at 5–6 years of age*

| | Low Birth Weight | | Control | | Test of Proportion |
|---|---|---|---|---|---|
| | 162 | | 109 | | |
| I.Q. | No | % | No | % | p value |
| ≤90 | 56 | 34.5 | 14 | 12.8 | <0.01 |
| 91–110 | 95 | 58.6 | 67 | 61.4 | >0.05 |
| 110 | 11 | 6.7 | 28 | 25.6 | <0.01 |

*Source:* Author.

**Table 2.3.14:**
*Mean IQ Levels in preterm AGA, term small for gestation, and cohort subjects at 5–6 years of age*

| | SMS | | | CIE | | | CD | | |
|---|---|---|---|---|---|---|---|---|---|
| Group | No. | Mean | p Value | No. | Mean | p Value | No. | Mean | p Value |
| Preterm AGA & Control | 40 | 97.59 | <.001 | 35 | 95.9 | <.05 | 17 | 95.9 | N.S. |
| Term Small for Gestation & Control | 37 | 100.7 | <.01 | 46 | 96.9 | <.05 | 14 | 105.1 | N.S. |

*Source:* Author.

disease. He suggested that foetal undernutrition at critical periods of development in utero and during infancy leads to permanent changes in body structure and metabolism. These changes result in increased adult susceptibility to coronary heart disease (CHD) and noninsulin-dependent diabetes mellitus (NIDDM). The publication by Professor Barker evoked tremendous interest at national and international levels. Numerous publications have been made describing the foetal growth deprivation effect on body composition, body metabolism, immune system, and systemic effects on body organs and functions, life cycles, and even the next generation.

The NDBC became associated with Professor Barker and his group to investigate his hypothesis and confirm or deny it in Indian subjects. The association began in 1995 and still continues with his group of workers at Medical Research Council (MRC), Southampton, even though Professor Barker passed away in 2013. We have investigated body growth from childhood to adulthood and its influence on metabolic diseases, cardiovascular system (CVS) effects, human capital development, intergeneration changes, and so forth. These data will be elaborated upon in later chapters in the second part of this book, which has been called the adult period of the NDBC.

## The Life Course of the NDBC Low Birth Wight Infants

The NDBC was founded to investigate the extent, nature, and immediate and long-term consequences of LBW infants. LBW has remained a focus throughout the NDBC studies from 1969 to 2015. The causes, mortality, morbidity, growth and development, and association with adult diseases have been described in detail elsewhere in this book. We were fortunate to have a life course of the NDBC from their birth through childhood, adolescence, and as a young adult to 46 years of age. We, therefore, analysed this life cycle for selected outcomes as it was not possible to do every aspect of the study in which the NDBC group was interested (Table 2.3.15).

### Education

Information was available for 271 which revealed that more than 50% of them were graduates or more. Only one subject was illiterate, primary and middle class education was seen in about 10%, and the remaining were high school or more. It seems the level of education was not affected by being born LBW with almost 100% literacy, more than 50% graduates, and about 10% of these being professionals.

**Table 2.3.15:**
*Life course of LBW in cohort subjects*

| | Low Birth Weight <2,500g (n=1,783) | | Normal Birth Weight ≥2,500g (n=5,055) | | P Value |
|---|---|---|---|---|---|
| | *n* | *%* | *n* | | |
| **Education** | | | | | |
| Illiterate | 271 | 0.4 | 898 | 0.4 | 0.552 |
| Primary school | | 4.1 | | 2.0 | |
| Middle school | | 5.5 | | 6.6 | |
| High school certificate | | 14.8 | | 14.5 | |
| High school+ | | 19.6 | | 17.4 | |
| Other graduate | | 44.6 | | 47.0 | |
| Professional degree | | 11.1 | | 12.1 | |
| **Occupation** | | | | | |
| Homemaker | 271 | 28.8 | 898 | 26.7 | 0.362 |
| Unemployed | | 0.7 | | 1.0 | |
| Unskilled manual, landless labour | | 1.8 | | 0.9 | |
| Semi-skilled manual labour, Marginal landowner, Rickshaw driver, army *jawan*, carpenter, fitter | | 8.5 | | 7.1 | |
| Skilled manual labour, small business owner, small farmer | | 18.8 | | 15.7 | |
| Trained, clerical, medium business owner, middle level farmer, teacher, maintenance (in charge), personal manager | | 32.8 | | 36.3 | |
| Professional, big business, landlord, university teacher, Class-I, IAS/ services, officer, lawyer | | 8.1 | | 11.1 | |
| Others | | 0.4 | | 1.1 | |
| **Stunting*** | | | | | |
| Birth | 1,713 | 37.2 | 4,923 | 3.1 | <0.001 |
| 6 months | 1,578 | 39.2 | 4,680 | 12.2 | <0.001 |
| 12 months | 1,172 | 54.3 | 3,637 | 27.0 | <0.001 |
| 24 months | 1,165 | 65.8 | 3,694 | 39.8 | <0.001 |
| 36 months | 1,115 | 67.2 | 3,545 | 42.7 | <0.001 |
| 48 months | 1,054 | 60.8 | 3,363 | 39.7 | <0.001 |
| 60 months | 919 | 52.9 | 3,020 | 34.2 | <0.001 |

| | Low Birth Weight <2,500g (n=1,783) | | Normal Birth Weight ≥2,500g (n=5,055) | | P Value |
|---|---|---|---|---|---|
| | n | % | n | | |
| ***Underweight#*** | | | | | |
| Birth | 1,764 | 71.8 | 5,043 | 0.0 | <0.001 |
| 6 months | 1,584 | 49.2 | 4,686 | 15.4 | <0.001 |
| 12 months | 1,173 | 42.7 | 3,642 | 17.8 | <0.001 |
| 24 months | 1,165 | 50.6 | 3,667 | 23.5 | <0.001 |
| 36 months | 1,109 | 45.8 | 3,522 | 21.9 | <0.001 |
| 48 months | 1,049 | 39.3 | 3,349 | 18.6 | <0.001 |
| 60 months | 921 | 37.9 | 3,026 | 17.6 | <0.001 |
| ***Wasting^*** | | | | | |
| Birth | 1,340 | 49.0 | 4,854 | 9.6 | <0.001 |
| 6 months | 1,580 | 23.3 | 4,677 | 9.2 | <0.001 |
| 12 months | 1,171 | 17.8 | 3,631 | 8.1 | <0.001 |
| 24 months | 1,162 | 16.0 | 3,658 | 6.9 | <0.001 |
| 36 months | 1,110 | 8.4 | 3,518 | 3.7 | <0.001 |
| 48 months | 1,046 | 6.4 | 3,344 | 2.2 | <0.001 |
| 60 months | 918 | 5.6 | 3,016 | 2.5 | <0.001 |
| **Gestation (weeks)** | | | | | |
| Preterm (<37) | 1,562 | 21.9 | 4,489 | 11.5 | <0.001 |
| Term (37–41) | | 68.1 | | 75.3 | |
| Post-term (≥41) | | 10.1 | | 13.2 | |
| Hypertension[a] | 349 | 26.6 | 1,156 | 26.0 | 0.835 |
| Diabetes[b] | 345 | 14.5 | 1,145 | 11.9 | 0.195 |
| Hypercholesterolaemia[c] | 344 | 56.4 | 1,145 | 54.8 | 0.621 |
| High triglyceride[d] | 344 | 44.5 | 1,145 | 42.5 | 0.535 |

**Source:** Author.

**Notes:** * Stunting-WHO height for age <–2.

\# Underweight-WHO weight for age <–2.

^ Wasting-WHO weight for height <–2.

[a] Hypertension was defined as systolic >=140 or diastolic >=90 or on anti-hypertensive medication.

[b] Diabetic was defined as fasting glucose >=126 mg/dl (7.0 mmol/l) or 120 min glucose >=200 mg/dl (11.1 mmol/l) or taking medicine(s) for diabetes.

[c] Hypercholesterolaemia was defined as fasting cholesterol >=5.2 mmol/l.

[d] High triglycerides was defined as serum triglyceride >=150 mg/dl.

*Occupation*

It showed a very wide range of employment amongst the LBW cohort with 40% of them being well employed. They were in service as clerks, teachers in schools and university, owned small or large business and some were farmers.

About 40% of the cohorts were homemakers, 12.88% were skilled worker, and remaining were semi-skilled manual workers, marginal landowners, and had miscellaneous occupation. Only 2.0% were unemployed. It seemed that the birth weight did not influence the occupation and perhaps they found employment as per their skills, education, and experience.

*Nutrition*

Nutritional status was available in large numbers until the age of 5 years. The numbers declined with increase in age, but still a significant numbers were available for assessment. We largely focused on undernutrition as the problem of overweight or obesity seemed to be negligible. LBW seemed to be prone to undernutrition as per the WHO criterion. A significant number of these children suffered with stunting, underweight, and wasting. Stunting was a major problem and seen through the first 5 years with its maximum occurrence in the crucial 2–3 years. About 40% were underweight at 5 years. Wasting decreased with increase in age from birth to 5 years. It is difficult to interpret the significance of these findings as LBW children in this study were mostly IUGR and growth retarded from birth. They remained thin and were at risk of developing cardiometabolic diseases in adult life if they put on weight beyond their potential.

## Chronic Adult Diseases

An alarming number of surviving LBW children developed adult diseases. The most common were high cholesterol (56.4%) and high triglyceride (44.5%). Hypertension was seen in 1/4th[th] or 26.6% and diabetes in 14.5% (Table 2.3.15). This study did not find any significant differences between LBW and normal children. This may be due to small numbers of LBW children and a larger study may show different results.

# 4

# Child Survival, Health, and Disease

## Breastfeeding Practices in Cohort

Infant feeding practices were studied in 802 randomly selected mothers of children over 1 year of age. The sample was representative of cross-cultural, economic, and ethnic groups. Breastfeeding was almost universal but for varying durations. About 5.5%, 11.7%, and 22.8% of the children were breastfed for less than 1 month, 2 months, and 6 months respectively. Literate and older mothers tended to breastfeed for shorter periods. Illiterate mothers, on the other hand, tended to prolong breastfeeding unduly. The sex of the infant and the duration of the urban stay of the mother did not seem to affect the duration of breastfeeding. Supplementation with liquid feeds, 50% diluted buffalo milk in the majority of cases, was begun rather early, but the introduction of semi-solids and solids was very often unduly delayed. This was particularly true among illiterate mothers. Thus, it is felt that a concerted effort to educate mothers, especially illiterate and under-privileged mothers, regarding the role of breastfeeding and the benefits of supplementation feeding would improve infant nutritional status [48].

## Cohort Child Mortality

Child mortality has always been one of the most challenging problems faced globally for many centuries. It is often considered as an index of country's development. In last 200 years, it was so high that even in the well-developed countries, every third child died. In India, the situation was worse and every second child died before reaching 5 years of age.

The leading causes of deaths were infections, especially with LBW and undernutrition as underlying factors.

The NDBC studies were launched in between 1969 and 1973, and at that time the under-five child mortality in India was still very high. The decline in under-five mortality globally has been striking, and currently globally only 3.47% of children die by 5 years of age. Some countries, including China, have rates which are even lower than this. In India, the scene is still dismal. The under-five mortality continues to be high after an initial sharp decline from 125.6 in 1990 to 61.2 in 2010, but the decline is now slow. This striking fall was perhaps due to decline in mortality from 1 month to 4 years of age, but not so in the neonatal mortality.

Survival as an outcome was a major objective of the NDBC. We were particularly interested in the mortality pattern, especially in the first 5 years of life. It is the most vulnerable period in childhood and the most critical days in this period are the first 28 days of life or the newborn period. Nearly 1/2 to 2/3rd of the under-five mortality occurs in the newborn period.

The total number of deaths in the NDBC was 401 during the first 5 years of life. The distribution of these by age periods is given in Table 2.4.1. The maximum number of deaths occurred in the first year with equal number in neonatal period and post-neonatal period of infancy. The mortality declined with increase in age and dropped to 1/4th the number in the second year, then to 1/3rd of the second year in the third year, and to 1/3rd to 2/3rd thereafter. The overall under-five mortality was 4.9 % (Table 2.4.1).

## Newborn Mortality

Newborn period is the one which extends from birth to 28 days of life. It is usually divided into two periods: the early neonatal period which covers 0–7 days of life and the late neonatal period which extends from 8–28 days of life. The periods have been divided because the morbidity and mortality in the two are distinct and need different kinds of strategies to deal with them as compared to later age periods.

**Table 2.4.1:**
*Mortality among cohort subjects from 0–5 years of age*

| Mortality Period | Number | Percent |
|---|---|---|
| Neonatal (birth–28 days) | 168 | 41.8 |
| Infant (29 days–1 yr) | 167 | 41.7 |
| 1–2 yrs | 37 | 9.3 |
| 2–3 yrs | 13 | 3.3 |
| 3–4 yrs | 7 | 1.7 |
| 4–5 yrs | 9 | 2.2 |
| **Total** | **401** | **100.0** |

*Source:* Author.

Mortality in newborns has remained a challenge from the last century and is currently the foremost challenge being faced at the global and national levels. The importance and relevance became increasingly evident with sharp and effective decline in under-five and infant mortality, but not a dramatic or as sharp a decline in neonatal mortality. For the past few decades, the attention of health providers and policy-makers has been on the newborn. Globally, the neonatal mortality fell by 40% in the last 20 years and the number of deaths fell from 4.7 million to 2.8 million. In India, the estimated neonatal deaths in 2013–14 have been over 0.5 million. The total number of deaths has indeed decreased sharply but this is still far from satisfactory [47, 49, 50].

In the NDBC, in 1969–73, the neonatal mortality was 24.9 per 1,000 live birth. Of this, 14.4 were early neonatal deaths (death from 0 to 8 days) and the remaining late neonatal deaths (age 8 to 28 days). In comparison to current national statistics it is still low as it still varies from 22.9 to 36.6 in different parts of the country. However, in the state of Delhi it is 14 and is significantly low after almost 40 years. The low mortality rate could be due to selection of the cohort, the general living conditions, family and maternal education, income level, pregravid maternal health, pregnancy and delivery care, and neonatal factors like birth weight [(52,53].

The major causes of neonatal deaths in the NDBC were preterm and LBW, which appeared to contribute directly or indirectly to neonatal mortality. The maternal age of less than 20 years and more than 40 years, primi and grand multi-parity appeared to be the other causes. Poor parental education, income, and living conditions further contributed to the mortality. The direct causes of deaths included asphyxia, respiratory distress, infections, and congenital malformations. Even now, at the national level, the causes remain the same with preterm, birth asphyxia, infections, and pneumonia being the foremost contributors to newborn mortality [49–51].

## Infant Mortality

In the 20th century, infant mortality was one of the most important child health key indices for measuring a country's health and health delivery system. It is defined as the number of deaths of infants under 1 year of age in a given year per 1,000 live births. It includes the total death rate and deaths of both sexes. In India, the present infant mortality rate is 42 [49,50].

In the NDBC, during the period 1969–73, the infant mortality was 46.50 and was largely contributed by a neonatal mortality of 21.18 per 1,000 births. It was high but was almost half as compared to the prevalent national infant mortality rate. The family profile contributing to the infant mortality was the continuation of neonatal factors and included others such as socio-economic and educational status, housing, and living conditions. The social factors were age at marriage, maternal educational status, and family conditions. The maternal biological factors were age, pre-pregnancy weight, height, and nutritional status. The pregnancy factors were parity, spacing between two successive pregnancies, and previous foetal or neonatal or child deaths. The infant causes included gender, birth weight, gestation, nutrition, and utilization of health care facilities. In twin births, the infant mortality was almost seven times as compared to single births [51–54].

## Under-five Mortality

The under-five mortality in the NDBC during the year 1969–73 was 43 per 1,000 live births. At this time, the focus of child mortality was on infant mortality. Under-five mortality as a measure of health became popular in the 1970s when David Morley introduced the health cards and under-five clinics. In the last two decades, under-five mortality has dropped by almost 47%. In India, the under-five mortality has also declined substantially but the decline has been slower than expected. The decline has largely resulted from decrease in deaths in newborns and mortality due to infectious diseases. In the developed countries, as also in almost all countries, the decline was also helped by improvement in health care and preventive methods in the health delivery system. As mentioned earlier, infant and neonatal mortality decline after an initial rapid phase has been somewhat slower. Currently, the neonatal mortality rate is 29, infant mortality rate 42, and under-five mortality 56.3 at the national level [49–51]. However, the child mortality rates vary from state to state, that is, in the state of Kerala it is 14 but in the in some states such as Madhya Pradesh, Bihar, and Rajasthan it varies between 70 and 90 [49–51].

The major causes that contribute to under-five mortality are LBW including extreme preterm and SGA births. A comparison of mortality rates between LBW <2,500 g and ≥2,500 g is given in Table 2.4.2 to show the influence of birth weight on under-five mortality rate. The direct causes of death recorded were birth asphyxia, infections, pneumonias, diarrhoea, malaria, measles, and childhood undernutrition. In the NDBC, apart from the listed causes, poor income, living conditions, sanitation, and maternal education were the other contributory factors.

## Cohort Morbidity

The morbidity follow-up was not specifically planned. It was recorded on a preset pro forma for children on recall basis by the family member. It was possible to assess 1,326 children of the available cohort; majority of these children were clinically normal with some aberrations/abnormality in few children. The liver was palpable in 60% and spleen in 4.5%. Amongst these, in 2%, the liver and spleen appeared to be abnormal. The cause for either spleen or liver enlargement was not available and these were identified on routine clinical examination.

The commonest morbidity was Pica or a disease characterized by eating dirt, hair, chalks, clothes paper, stone, etc. Amongst infections, acute or recurrent diarrhoea appeared to be the most common. Acute or chronic diarrhoea was seen in 13.05%. The other morbidity commonly seen was respiratory infections such as pneumonia/bronchitis in about 12%. Measles-like illness was also reported in 12% and whooping cough in 3.5% of the children. Other morbidities were ear discharge in

**Table 2.4.2:**
*Perinatal and under-five mortality in cohort subjects with birth weight <2,500 g (LBW) and ≥2,500 g*

| Mortality Period | N | Low Birth Weight (<2,500 g) | Birth Weight ≥2,500 g |
|---|---|---|---|
| Perinatal (28 weeks gestation – 7 days) | 50 | 70.0 | 30.0 |
| Neonatal (8 days – 28 days) | 43 | 76.7 | 23.3 |
| Infant (29 days – 1 yr) | 117 | 53.0 | 47.0 |
| 1–2 yrs | 27 | 33.3 | 66.7 |
| 2–3 yrs | 11 | 45.5 | 54.5 |
| 3–4 yrs | 7 | 57.1 | 42.9 |
| 4–5 yrs | 9 | 22.2 | 77.8 |

| Mortality Period | N | Gestation (weeks) <37 | ≥37 |
|---|---|---|---|
| Perinatal (28 weeks gestation – 7 days) | 104 | 43.3 | 56.7 |
| Neonatal (8 days – 28 days) | 55 | 43.6 | 56.4 |
| Infant (29 days – 1 yr) | 127 | 24.4 | 75.6 |
| 1–2 yrs | 23 | 13.0 | 87.0 |
| 2–3 yrs | 11 | 45.5 | 54.5 |
| 3–4 yrs | 7 | 14.3 | 85.7 |
| 4–5 yrs | 5 | 0.0 | 100.0 |

*Source:* Author.

9% and accidents including burns in 1.4%. Acute and chronic diarrhoea and infections as common morbidities is consistent with the findings of similar studies. However, pica and ear infections have not been so commonly reported. Measles and whooping cough were quite prevalent as the immunization status of the children was poor [54].

## Congenital Malformations

Congenital anomalies can be defined as structural or functional anomalies (e.g., metabolic disorders) that occur during intrauterine life and can be identified prenatally, at birth or later in life. Estimating the prevalence of congenital malformations was one of the main initial objectives. As per WHO classification for congenital malformations, the prevalence of major and minor malformations in infants who could be examined was 26.22 per 1,000 births. Of these, 11.07 were major and the remaining were minor. At birth, anomalies of musculo-skeletal system were the most common at 7.38 per 1,000 births. These were followed by the central nervous system in 3.16, genito-urinary in 2.5, gastro intestinal in 1.98, and cardiovascular in 1.45 per thousand births. Anomalies of skin and its appendages were the most frequent minor anomalies. The prevalence of malformations in the cohort is not unusual as ultrasound assessments were not available and prenatal folic acid administration was not in vogue at that time. The prevalence is similar to that reported in community-based study but less in comparison to the hospital-based cohort or follow-up study. No specific cause could be ascribed to this difference but it may be related to occurrence of high risk deliveries at hospital and to better education, nutrition, and antenatal care in the cohort as compared to hospital births. This may also be due to less searching questions or the lack of investigations and medical follow-up [55, 56].

## Immunization

Small pox vaccine was the most commonly administered and accepted immunization. It was confirmed with the presence of a scar in 95.4% of children. Diphtheria, pertussis, and tetanus (DPT) and polio immunization with recommended and three doses was recorded in 54.8% and 60.9%, respectively. About 75% of the infants received DPT and polio in the first year and 5.8% in the second year. Bacille Calmette Guerin (BCG) at birth was given in only 35.5% of the children even though more than 2/3rds of deliveries were institution or facility based.

The immunization status was significantly influenced if the birth occurred in a health care facility or at home. This was true irrespective of births occurring in a private or government hospital, nursing home or maternal and child health centre, or at home. Thus, small pox vaccination coverage was 99.2% in a private nursing home as against 94–96% at home or at a government hospital. The differences were more significant for DPT, polio, and BCG if the birth occurred in a health facility as against home. For polio, the vaccination rate was 70% for facility-based delivery as against 39.6% for home. For DPT, it was 66–70% for facility based as against 29.5% for home. For BCG, it was dismal (7.3%) for home births as against 50–56% in institutional/facility-based birth.

Maternal literacy also had a direct influence on successful immunization rates for the primary vaccination of BCG, small pox, DPT, and polio. Socio-economic status as assessed by per capita income also positively affected the vaccination rate. It increased almost sevenfold for BCG from the lowest income of ₹20 per month to ₹301 or more. Similarly, DPT and polio successful immunization rates almost doubled from the lowest income to highest income groups [57].

PART 3

# Growth, Cognitive Development, and Nutrition

# 1

# Growth

## Introduction

In the 1960s, there was hardly any reference or standard for body growth measurements relating to weight, height, and head circumference for children of our population. It is known that growth standards and patterns differ from country to country, within the country, and in different communities. India is a large country with a current population of over 1.2 billion, 29 states, urban and rural population, and numerous castes, customs, faiths, and beliefs. Our country which was enslaved for centuries and deprived of education and remained seeped in poverty is bound to have growth patterns which are different from the ones available in the literature from different countries. There were occasional Indian studies which were being referred to as reference for the Indian children. We, therefore, accorded high priority to physical growth of the children so as to develop reference standards from a representative urban population through a well-designed, prospective age-specific, body growth study.

## Study Sample, Methods, and Techniques

The NDBC initially had a sample of 8,181 children as cohort. The follow-up of children over a 20-year study period resulted in loss to follow-up at different points of time and at different ages. Thus, from an initial sample of 8,181 children we were able to study growth in 1,092 children who had attained the age of 20 years and were available for follow-up.

The measurements were recorded by trained anthropologists after a medical examination by a medical officer. All children with acute problems or those with conditions likely to affect growth were excluded. If the measurement date on a child was missed, the measurements obtained at that time were excluded from analysis.

## Growth Measurements

The measurements for growth studies were obtained initially for weight, length/height, and head circumference. But later on, additional measurements of mid-arm circumference, chest circumference, and sitting height were also added. In the first year of life, the measurements were obtained at 3-month intervals and within a week's time, and thereafter every 6 months and within 2 weeks of the expected measurements date till 20 years of age. Standard techniques for recording measurements as described earlier were used.

## Analysis

The analysis of the body measurement at different age point was done by calculating means and SD, growth percentiles, and Z scores using standard statistical tests. The percentiles commonly known as centile is a measure used in statistics to indicate the value below which a certain ranked child in a group of observations will fall. For example, a third centile for height represents a subject who would be ranked third among 100 subjects arranged in ascending order of their stature. Thus, the growth curves help in delineating the position of an individual on a given reference distribution. Children measuring between 3rd and 97th centile are considered to be within the normal range and those below 3rd centile or above 97th centile as below normal and above normal, respectively.

The Z scores are expressed in terms of SDs from their means. The Z scores have a distribution with a mean of 0 and SD of 1. It is calculated as

*Z-score (or SD-score)=(observed value–median value of the reference population)/standard deviation value of reference population*

The measurements obtained between –2 SD and +2 SD value of Z scores are regarded as normal, those below –2 SD as underweight, and those below –3 SD as severe underweight. Those above +2 SD are regarded as overweight.

## Interpretation of Growth Parameters

### Weight for Age

This is a measure of the child which is compared with a reference standard of similar age and gender. When the Z score is below –2 SD, it is underweight; and if it is below –3 SD, it is severely underweight.

### Weight for Length/Height

This is a measure of weight for a given length/height (irrespective of age) in comparison to the reference standards. A child with a weight for a given length/height, which is below –2 Z score is labelled as wasted (pathologically thin), while the one below –3 Z score is severely wasted.

### Length/Height for Age

It is a measure of the height of a child and needs to be compared to length/height of a reference standard for the same age and sex. A child with –2 Z score heights is stunted (pathologically short), and the one with –3 Z score is severely stunted.

The growth standard reference charts commonly used are of WHO (MGRS) and the Indian Academy of Paediatrics (IAP) growth charts of 2015.

## Body Mass Index

It is computed as kg of body weight per height in meters squared (m²; BMI = weight in kg/height in m²). The BMI for children is variable with age as a child is continuously growing. BMI percentile curves are used for defining overweight and obesity. Different cut-offs have been suggested by the International Obesity Task Force and various Indian workers.

## Physical Growth

A child continues to grow physically, emotionally, intellectually, and sexually till adulthood. For convenience and for logistic reasons, the child's age is divided into different periods, namely, early childhood period (0–2 years) including infancy (up to one year), two to five years, 6–10 years, and adolescence (10–19 years). The first 2 years are most critical years for survival and sequelae in immediate and later life. In this period, there is rapid body growth and most of the brain grows during this period. The factors affecting growth may also influence brain development. It has also been shown that growth in this period may influence adult human capital development including educational attainment, income earning capacity, stature, and even the birth weight of the next offspring.

The growth slows between 3 and 5 years of age and is the slowest in mid-childhood. It again accelerates and is rapid with the onset of adolescence when the child matures into an adult. During adolescence, a lot of hormonal influences affect body, reproductive, and emotional growth. In view of the physiological, physical, and endocrinal changes and susceptibilities to morbidities, we analysed the growth of the cohort from childhood to adulthood in different age periods, namely, birth to five years, five years to ten years, and 11 to 19 years and also as a composite growth curve from birth to 20 years of age.

### Growth from Birth to Five Years

This period is considered to be the most vulnerable period of childhood. During this period, the child is most susceptible to illnesses which may be minor, recurrent, or serious enough to effect growth or even endanger life. The most common illnesses affecting growth are infections and nutritional disorders.

Growth is fastest in the first 3 months: the child grows at 20–30 g per day. It then slows down during the rest of infancy period. The growth then further slows down in the second year to almost half the early growth as body nutritional needs decrease and physical activity increases. During 3–5 years, the child gains 2–2.5 kg and 6.0 cm per year. The NDBC children followed a similar pattern.

### Growth from 6 to 10 Years

Growth during 6–10 years continues to be slow and steady and is slowest for the entire childhood period. These are crucial years for growth monitoring as the child may continue to suffer from malnutrition due to under or overnutrition.

### Growth from 11 to 19 Years or in Adolescence

This period of growth is critical in human life. It is at this time that the body not only begins to attain the final shape in body size but also develops with respect to emotional, mental, and reproductive growth. Boys and girls follow a different pattern of growth due to biological changes occurring in the reproductive organs. The growth velocity at this time increases and almost doubles the pre-pubertal period of childhood.

The onset of growth is earlier in this period in the girls as compared to the boys. The girls show a peak in growth velocity, early onset of pubertal growth, and before occurrence of menarche or menstrual period. The body grows at about 9 cm in height per year. The development of breast buds marks the beginning of the pubertal growth. Menarche occurs around 9–12 years of age and 2–3 years after the onset of puberty in girls.

The boys' growth in this period usually starts 2–3 years later than girls at around 12–15 years of age. They grow at a faster rate than girls with a mean growth rate of 7–13 cm per year. Testicular enlargement marks the beginning of pubertal growth in boys.

## Growth from Birth to 20 Years

Linear growth curves from birth to adulthood provide its own advantages. It gives a peep into one's physical development over the crucial years of childhood growth and development. It helps identify periods of faltering, slow, and accelerated growth. It, thus, helps in identifying age-specific growth-related problems during the childhood to adulthood life course.

Growth studies in children have been a subject of interest, concern, and research for many decades. Several studies have been published, which report cross-sectional, semi-longitudinal, or mixed longitudinal data, but there were hardly any longitudinal studies from birth to adulthood from a well-defined urban community from our country. The NDBC study is a unique growth study from a representative urban community which has recorded growth from birth to 20 years at age-specific periods. It provides growth curves for means and SDs, percentiles, incremental or growth velocity, and Z scores. Some studies done during the comparable NDBC study period include the ICMR (1956–65) and Aggarwal et al. [58–60]. The ICMR study was a cross sectional study from a pooled national data with specific age known in only 25% of the children with mixed socio-economic status. The Aggarwal et al. study is also a cross-sectional, multicentre study from children of high income parents.

At the international level, there were many studies but the most often referred studies are of the NCHS and the Center for Disease Control and Prevention (CDC) from America and Tanner from UK. In 2006, WHO published growth norms (WHO MGRS) from a multi-country study from birth to five years from exclusively breastfed children for first the 6 months, and with other criteria for inclusion in the study. India was part of this six multi-country study [61]. The WHO has also developed standard growth charts from 6 to 18 years based on the original NCHS data of 1963–94. The other recent Indian studies are by Khadilkar [62]. But the most recent study is the *Growth Standard* published by the Indian Academy of Paediatrics from a multicentre study in 11 cities [62]. The growth pattern of the NDBC is given in Table 3.1.1 and its comparisons with IAP growth curves in Figures 3.1.1–3.1.4.

The growth pattern of the NDBC from 1969 to 1991 with the IAP 2015 growth data curves is compared in Figures 3.1.1–3.1.4. There is a striking difference between the two growth patterns. The NDBC children

**Table 3.1.1:**
*Body growth in weight from birth to 20 years in cohort subjects*

| *Age* | *Weight (kg)* | | *Height (cm)* | | *BMI (kg/m²)* | |
|---|---|---|---|---|---|---|
| *(years)* | *N* | *Mean (SD)* | *N* | *Mean (SD)* | *N* | *Mean (SD)* |
| Birth | 6,806 | 2.8 (0.4) | 6,641 | 48.3 (2.2) | 6,639 | 11.9 (1.3) |
| 0.5 | 6,872 | 6.7 (1.0) | 6,862 | 64.5 (2.7) | 6,858 | 16.0 (1.6) |
| 1 | 5,354 | 8.2 (1.2) | 5,351 | 71.1 (3.2) | 5,342 | 16.2 (1.5) |
| 2 | 5,295 | 10.1 (1.4) | 5,335 | 80.5 (3.9) | 5,282 | 15.6 (1.3) |
| 3 | 5,087 | 12.0 (1.6) | 5,119 | 88.1 (4.5) | 5,080 | 15.4 (1.3) |
| 4 | 4,802 | 13.7 (1.7) | 4,826 | 95.0 (4.6) | 4,794 | 15.2 (1.1) |
| 5 | 4,296 | 15.3 (1.9) | 4,289 | 101.5 (4.8) | 4,283 | 14.8 (1.1) |
| 6 | 4,132 | 16.7 (2.2) | 4,124 | 107.7 (5.2) | 4,120 | 14.4 (1.1) |
| 7 | 3,995 | 18.4 (2.5) | 3,987 | 113.6 (5.4) | 3,981 | 14.2 ()1.1 |
| 8 | 3,861 | 20.5 (3.1) | 3,850 | 119.2 (5.6) | 3,847 | 14.4 (1.3) |
| 9 | 3,601 | 22.8 (3.6) | 3,588 | 124.6 (5.9) | 3,587 | 14.6 (1.4) |
| 10 | 3,383 | 25.0 (4.0) | 3,373 | 129.6 (6.4) | 3,371 | 14.8 (1.5) |
| 11 | 3,254 | 28.4 (5.3) | 3,248 | 135.5 (6.8) | 3,245 | 15.4 (1.8) |
| 12 | 3,245 | 32.0 (6.6) | 3,239 | 141.3 (7.3) | 3,238 | 15.9 (2.2) |
| 13 | 3,237 | 36.4 (7.8) | 3,233 | 147.1 (7.7) | 3,233 | 16.7 (2.5) |
| 14 | 3,201 | 41.1 (8.3) | 3,197 | 152.7 (7.8) | 3,197 | 17.5 (2.7) |
| 15 | 3,072 | 45.6 (8.6) | 3,066 | 157.2 (8.1) | 3,066 | 18.4 (2.8) |
| 16 | 2,675 | 48.9 (9.0) | 2,675 | 159.9 (8.8) | 2,672 | 19.1 (3.0) |
| 17 | 1,698 | 51.0 (9.5) | 1,702 | 161.4 (9.3) | 1,697 | 19.5 (3.1) |
| 18 | 1,075 | 51.8 (10.3) | 1,075 | 161.8 (9.7) | 1,073 | 19.7 (3.1) |
| 19 | 995 | 53.2 (10.5) | 995 | 162.4 (9.5) | 994 | 20.1 (3.2) |

*Source:* Author.

are lighter in weight and smaller in height all along from 5 to 18 year of age. The difference in weight for boys at 18 years of age is 7 kg and for girls is 4.9 kg. The difference in height for boys is 4.1 cm and for girls 2.8 cm. The significantly better growth of IAP children reflects secular trends and is also because of better nutrition, health care, and environment and socio-economic changes which have occurred during the last 50 years in India.

**Figure 3. 1.1:**
*Comparison of NDBC and IAP percentile curves in weight for boys from 0 to 18 years*

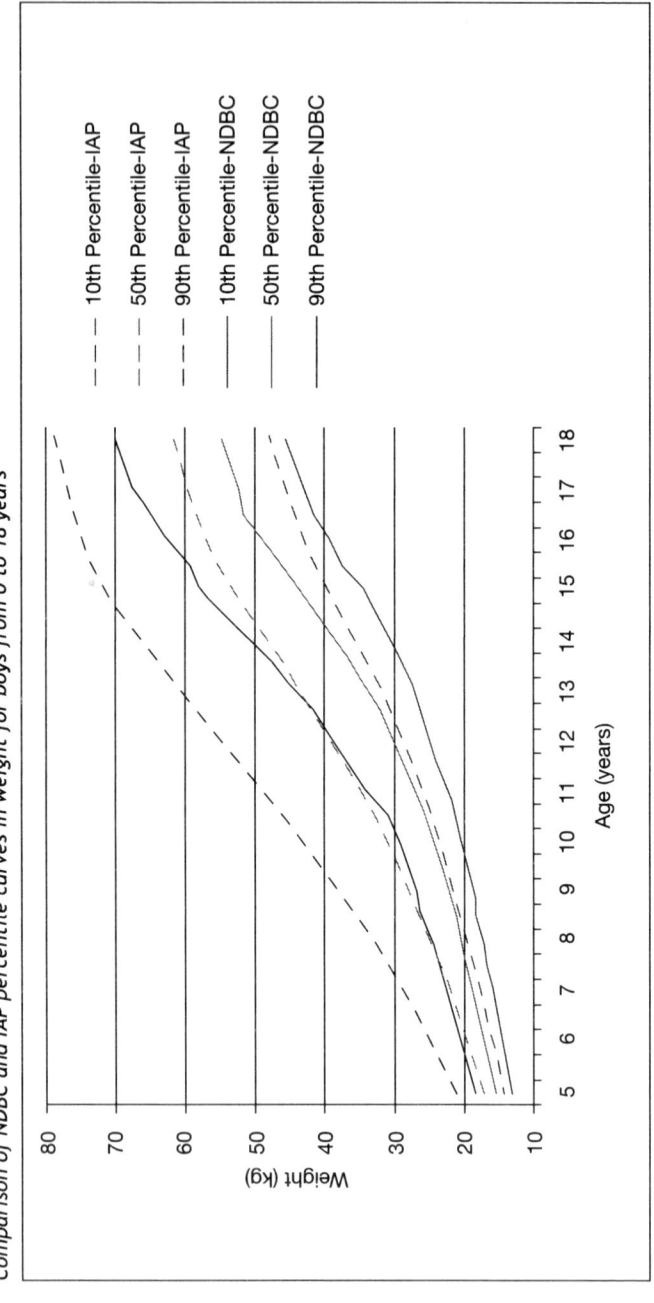

**Figure 3.1.2:**
*Comparison of NDBC and IAP percentile curves in weight for girls from 0 to 18 years*

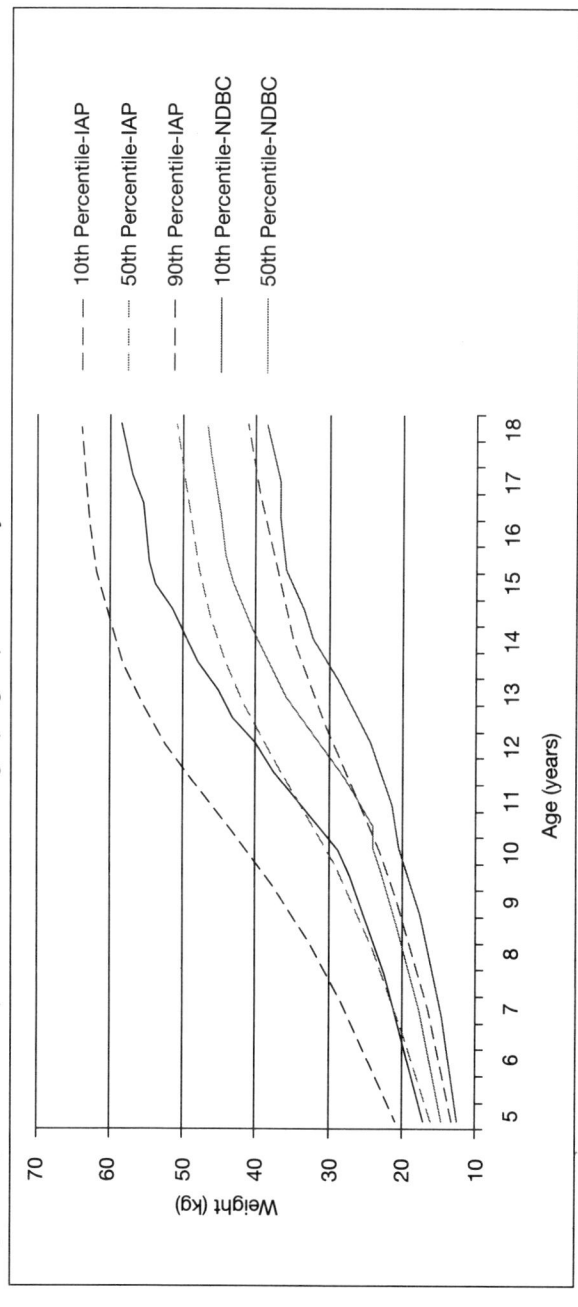

— — 10th Percentile-IAP
········· 50th Percentile-IAP
— — 90th Percentile-IAP
——— 10th Percentile-NDBC
········· 50th Percentile-NDBC

*Source:* Author.

**Figure 3.1.3:**
*Comparison of NDBC and IAP percentile curves in height for boys from 0 to 18 years*

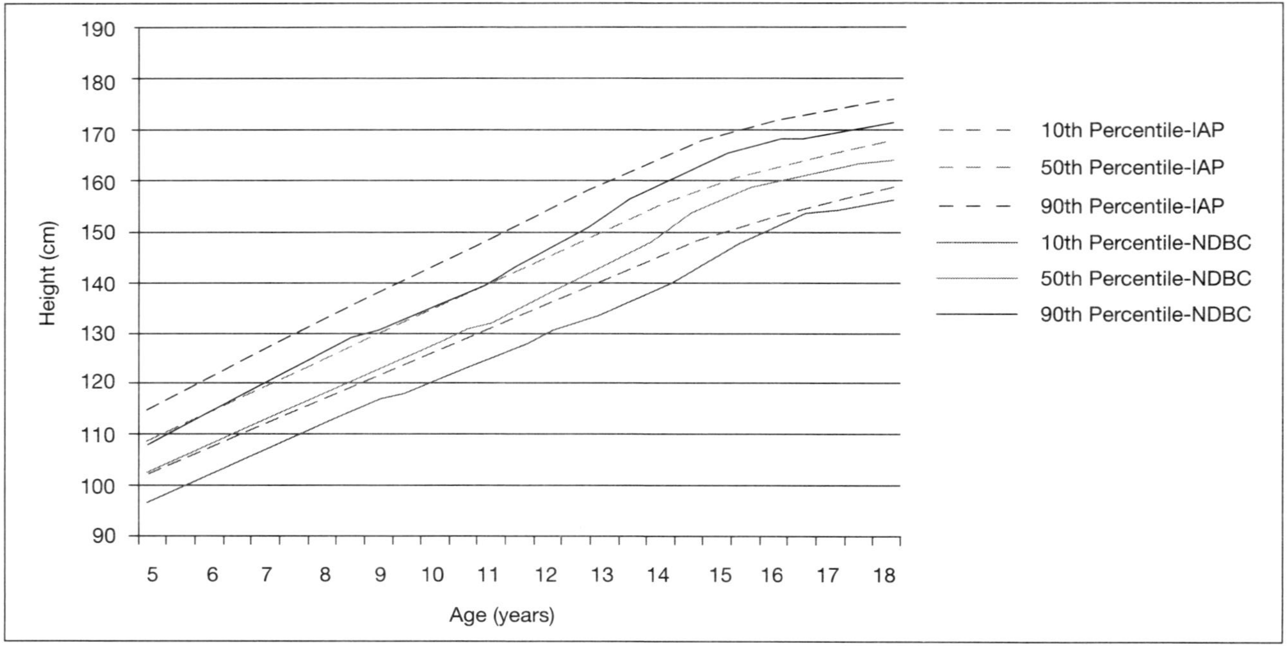

Height (cm)

Age (years)

- - - 10th Percentile-IAP
- - - 50th Percentile-IAP
- - - 90th Percentile-IAP
—— 10th Percentile-NDBC
—— 50th Percentile-NDBC
—— 90th Percentile-NDBC

*Source:* Author.

**Figure 3.1.4:**
*Comparison of NDBC and IAP percentile curves in height for girls from 0 to 18 years*

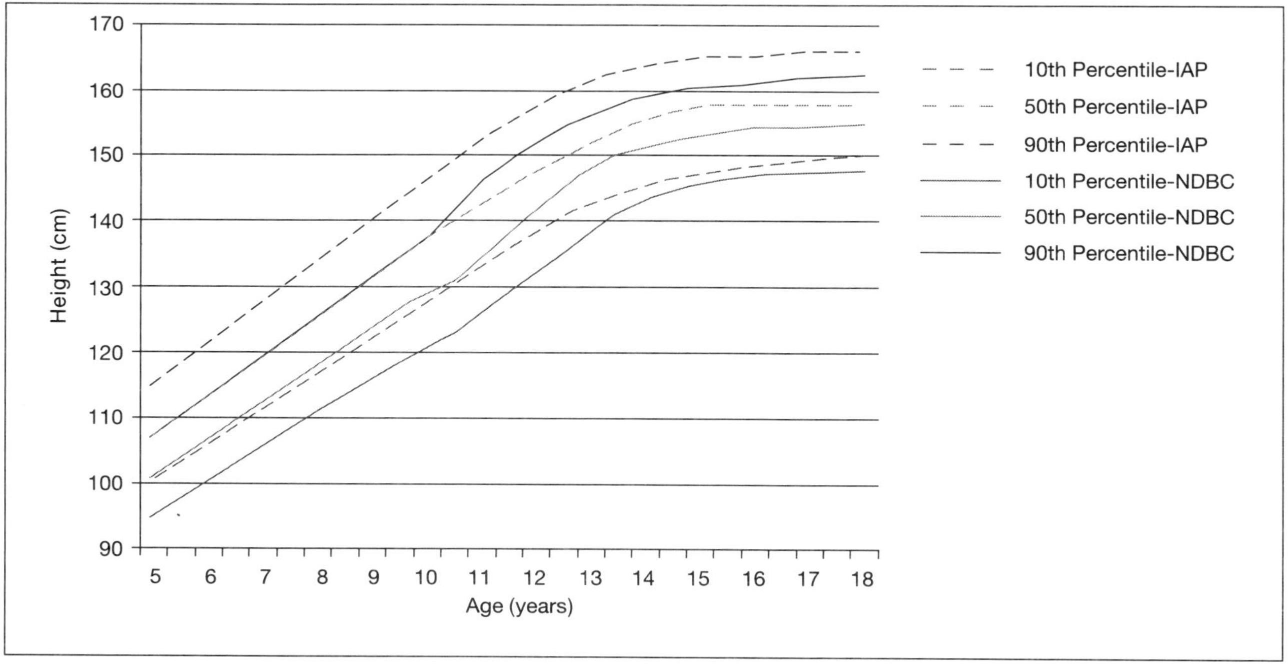

Legend:
- 10th Percentile-IAP
- 50th Percentile-IAP
- 90th Percentile-IAP
- 10th Percentile-NDBC
- 50th Percentile-NDBC
- 90th Percentile-NDBC

Height (cm): 90, 100, 110, 120, 130, 140, 150, 160, 170

Age (years): 5, 6, 7, 8, 9, 10, 11, 12, 13, 14, 15, 16, 17, 18

***Source:*** Author.

## Growth of Head Circumference

### Boys

The head growth of the NDBC showed a rapid increase in first year and gained almost 10 cm in size. It continued to grow in the second year by about 2 cm and thereafter at a very slow rate. It almost stopped growing by 13 years of age (54.2 cm) and measured 55 cm by age 19 years, when the growth stopped (Figure 3.1.5).

### Girls

The pattern of head growth for girls was similar to boys. It grew at a similar velocity but was smaller in measurement till adulthood. The NDBC head growth is comparable to other studies (Figure 3.1.6) [63, 64].

**Figure 3.1.5:**
*Growth in head circumference of NDBC from birth to 20 years*

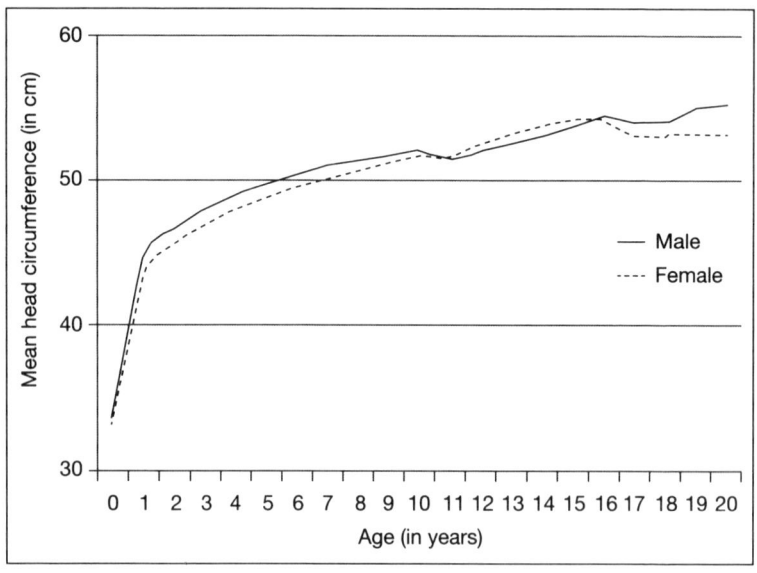

*Source:* Author.

**Figure 3.1.6:**
*Percentile growth in head circumference of NDBC from birth to 20 years*

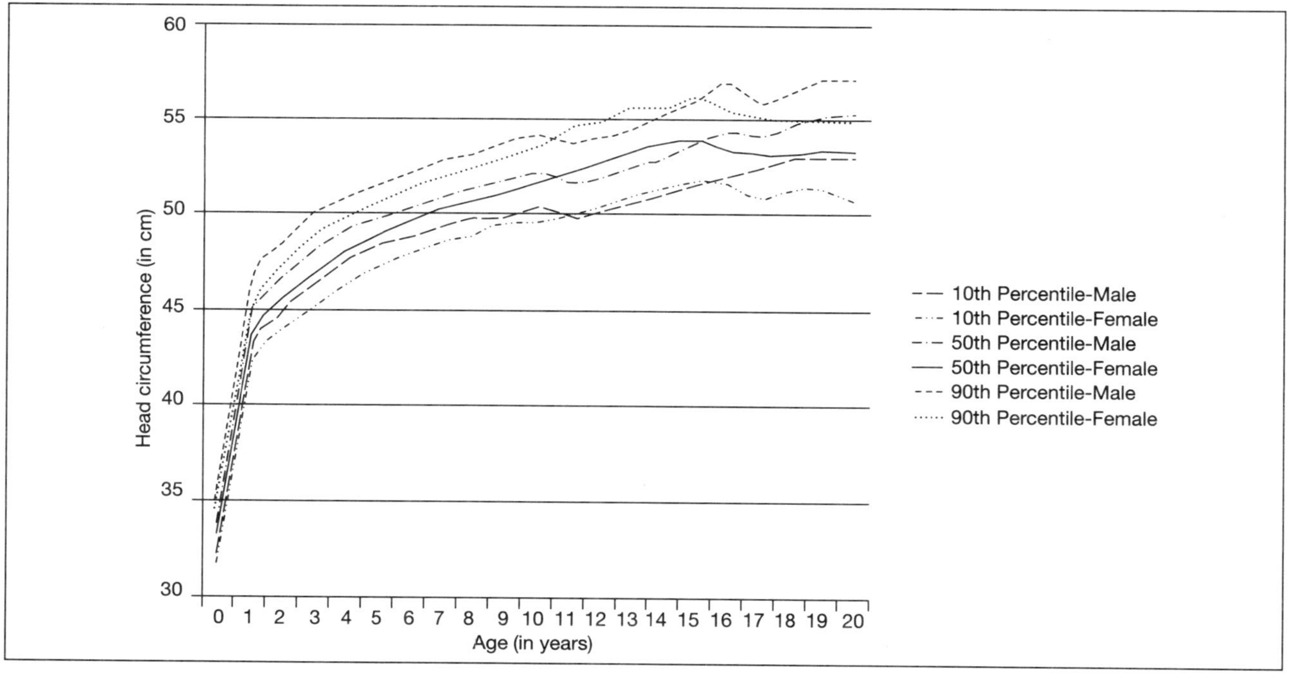

**Source:** Author.

## Z Score

The growth pattern is determined by calculating the mean Z scores for both boys and girls from birth to 19 years of age. The Z scores are primarily calculated to compare the growth with other studies. Currently in India, we have adopted the WHO Z scores from birth to five years and for 5–18 the Z scores of IAP have now become available. The other which is being used is of WHO which has been merged with old NCHS growth data.

The implications of Z scores growth data has been discussed in chapter on malnutrition, which elaborates undernutrition and overnutrition or obesity. The Z score for the NDBC is given in Table 3.1.2.

## Incremental Growth

The incremental growth is defined as the rate at which the growth occurs in certain periods. In the NDBC, growth rates were determined for every 3 months in first year and every 6 months thereafter. The rate of growth varied at different age periods. If the rate of growth was faster, the quantum of growth or gain in measurement was also higher, but if the rate of growth was slower than the quantum of growth was smaller.

The NDBC growth study had recorded the growth studies over a period and was age and time specific. Hence, we were able to construct the incremental growth curves from birth to 20 years which are described further.

### Incremental Growth Boys

The growth was rapid in the first 2 years, with maximum gains and rate occurring in the first 3 months of life. The boys gained about 2.4 kg in the first 3 months or about 26 g/day. It decreased to almost 15–20 g a day thereafter. The growth was slowest in mid childhood or 6–10 years of age. The pre-pubertal weight gain occurred from 12 years of age and continued till 15 years of age when it petered off.

The gains in height followed a similar pattern with a gain of 10.8 cm from birth length of 48.6 cm. The boys had attained about half their adult height between 2 and 2 ½ years of age when they measured

**Table 3.1.2:**
*Mean WHO anthropometric Z scores from birth to 20 years age of cohorts*

| Age (years) | Weight for Age | | Length/Height for Age | | BMI for Age | | Weight for Length | |
|---|---|---|---|---|---|---|---|---|
| | N | Mean (SD) | N | Mean (SD) | N | Mean (SD) | N | Mean (SD) |
| 0.5 | 6,867 | −1.22 (1.20) | 6,856 | −1.02 (1.17) | 6,846 | −0.85 (1.17) | 6853 | −0.69 (1.16) |
| 1 | 5,350 | −1.19 (1.21) | 5,347 | −1.54 (1.23) | 5,338 | −0.39 (1.15) | 5338 | −0.55 (1.14) |
| 2 | 5,295 | −1.44 (1.13) | 5,330 | −2.13 (1.22) | 5,283 | −0.11 (1.04) | 5283 | −0.45 (1.04) |
| 3 | 5,086 | −1.42 (1.04) | 5,112 | −1.99 (1.16) | 5,081 | −0.16 (0.98) | 5081 | −0.41 (0.96) |
| 4 | 4,802 | −1.35 (0.95) | 4,822 | −1.90 (1.06) | 4,794 | −0.14 (0.88) | 4794 | −0.30 (0.90) |
| 5 | 4,296 | −1.37 (0.89) | 4,288 | −1.74 (1.02) | 4,283 | −0.37 (0.80) | 4283 | −0.46 (0.83) |
| 6 | 4,132 | −1.54 (0.95) | 4,124 | −1.57 (1.02) | 4,120 | −0.74 (0.83) | — | — |
| 7 | 3,995 | −1.57 (0.99) | 3,987 | −1.43 (1.00) | 3,981 | −0.95 (0.86) | — | — |
| 8 | 3,861 | −1.55 (1.02) | 3,850 | −1.35 (0.98) | 3,847 | −1.01 (0.90) | — | — |
| 9 | 3,601 | −1.53 (1.02) | 3,588 | −1.31 (0.97) | 3,587 | −1.04 (0.93) | — | — |
| 10 | 3,383 | −1.60 (1.01) | 3,373 | −1.35 (1.02) | 3,370 | −1.15 (0.91) | — | — |
| 11 | — | — | 3,248 | −1.27 (1.05) | 3,244 | −1.14 (1.08) | — | — |
| 12 | — | — | 3,239 | −1.27 (1.05) | 3,235 | −1.17 (1.19) | — | — |
| 13 | — | — | 3,233 | −1.26 (1.06) | 3,231 | −1.13 (1.25) | — | — |
| 14 | — | — | 3,197 | −1.20 (1.05) | 3,195 | −1.03 (1.25) | — | — |
| 15 | — | — | 3,066 | −1.12 (0.99) | 3,066 | −0.89 (1.19) | — | — |
| 16 | — | — | 2,675 | −1.09 (0.93) | 2,672 | −0.79 (1.12) | — | — |
| 17 | — | — | 1,702 | −1.09 (0.89) | 1,696 | −0.78 (1.12) | — | — |
| 18 | — | — | 1,075 | −1.13 (0.91) | 1,073 | −0.84 (1.19) | — | — |
| 19 | — | — | 995 | −1.09 (0.93) | 994 | −0.81 (1.23) | — | — |

**Source:** Author.

**Figure 3.1.7:**
*Incremental growth in weight of NDBC from birth to 20 years*

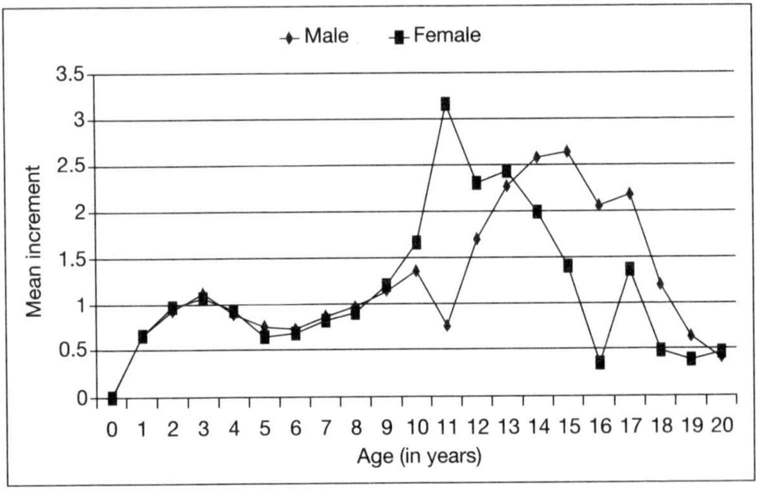

*Source:* Author.

between 85 and 89 cm compared to 155.2 cm at 19 years of age. The pubertal growth spurt was seen at 12 years, peaking at 14 years of age. It decelerated after that and the boys stopped growing after 19 years of age (Figure 3.1.7) [65].

### Incremental Growth Girls

The girls followed a pattern similar to boys but gain in weight was of smaller quantum and at a slower rate. They tripled their birth weight by 1 year of age and it slowed thereafter. However, the girls began to gain more than boys from 7 years of age and became heavier by 8 years. The weight reached its peak at 12 years and the rate of growth declined thereafter. The girls remained heavier than the boys from 9 to 12 years of age but weighed less after 13 years of age.

The height pattern was similar to the boys and followed them from birth till 10 years. At this age, the girls had a growth spurt in height and gained at a rapid rate as compared to boys, till 12–13 years of age. Thereafter, the growth velocity in height declined and the girls too stopped growing after the age of 19 years (Figure 3.1.8).

**Figure 3.1.8:**
*Incremental growths in height of NDBC from birth to 20 years*

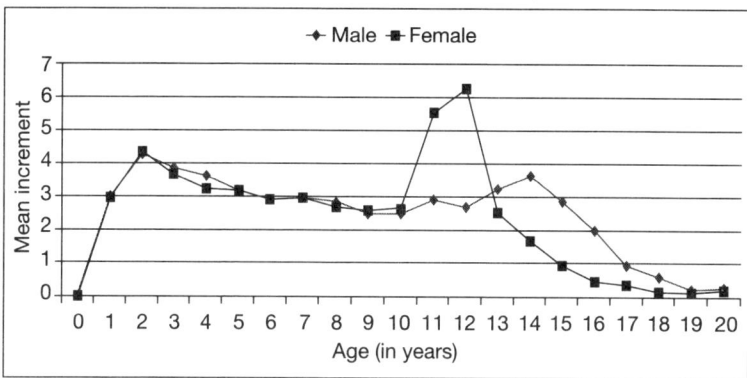

*Source:* Author.

# 2

# Cognitive Development

## Introduction

One of the major objectives of the study was to determine the influence of birth weight, specially the LBW group of ≤2,000 g, on child development. It was a difficult task to fulfil as developmental assessment is dependent on the application of an appropriate developmental scale, socio-economic and educational status of parents, and cultural practices, language, and communication amongst the families and community. This cohort was a spectrum of mixed population in terms of environment, family income, parental education, religion, social background, exposure to cultural practices, age at schooling, and other factors. Indian-children-specific, vernacular-, or regional-language-specific tests were not developed or tested and available at that period. The standard developmental scales such as the Gessels Developmental Scale (NCERT Adaption) [66–68] which was available had to be discarded because of non-availability of equipment and trained personnel. However, Indian versions (modified or adapted) were available and in use in developmental clinics and educational institutions. For this study, we used the intelligence tests which had been adapted by the Central Institute of Education (CIE), University of Delhi, as this was considered more appropriate and user friendly for the population [66].

## Subjects and Methods

The design of the NDBC cohort study permitted an investigation of the influence of parents' education, socio-economic status, family living conditions, employment of mother, exposure to preschooling, and gender on the CD of the children. It was also decided to test some selective independent and dependent variables respectively in children at age four and then at six years of the age and, hence, a set of dependent and independent variables for both age groups of the children were selected.

Every month, successively, 60 children were randomly selected from amongst the cohort children who were completing four years of age to provide a sample size of 50 subjects who were to be available by the time they completed six years of age. The ultimate objective was to have a sample size of 50 children in each batch of children after attrition due to drop out, lack of cooperation, shift out study area, and others.

The CIE individual scale of intelligence (CIE scale), which is a 1957 adaptation of Jerman–Merill's revision of the Stanford-Binnet [66] test, was selected for testing the CD in the cohort children. It has six items with two alternatives (6+2) for each age group from 3 to 11 years and six items each for 12 to 15 years of age. The details for its administration, scoring, and interpretation were readily available as per the test manual in use.

For CD testing of the children at six years of age, the subsets which were included in the development scales were block building, naming days and date, story comprehension, matching and naming of six colours, differences and similarities, opposite analogies, animal house, copying geometric design, missing features, and arithmetic problems.

The procedure of administering these tests involved a psychologist in a relaxed home environment so as to obtain optimum response and cooperation of children. The tests had to be performed in the presence of a family member for logistic reasons. The analysis was done after converting raw scores of the CD tests into percentages and appropriate statistical tests were applied for determining significance.

A total of 1,059 children were assessed on different tests. The same children were followed again at six years of age. Several sessions had to be done on the same child. Each session usually lasted 30–45 minutes. The responses were duly recorded on a pretested pro forma and the scores were calculated.

## Observations

Two distinct patterns influencing CD were observed. The first one related to the educational status of the parents and the other to the preschool exposure. The preschool going children scored higher at four years, but the difference seemed to disappear at 6 years as almost all children were attending school by six years of age.

Mother's and father's education directly influenced the IQ scores. Similarly, parental income also had a positive influence on IQ scores. However, the most significant influencing factor seemed to be attendance at the preschool, which even out-weighed parental income and maternal education.

Mother's employment status affected cognitive scores. Children whose mothers worked outside seemed to perform better and scored higher on IQ scales.

The number of siblings similarly also affected the scores. Children with three or less siblings had better scores then those with four or more siblings. The number of rooms in the residence affected the scoring in older children at six years of age. The sex of the child did not seem to influence the IQ scores but the first-born children scored better than those who were fourth or more in birth order. It was observed that the children of low socio-economic status performed poorly as compared to those who were from higher income levels.

The differential performance of the children could also be due to their familiarity with testing materials or testing situations as evident from the results of the present study. Children who had attended preschool, irrespective of which socio-economic status they belonged to, scored significantly higher at all levels than the ones who had not, thereby indicating positive transfer effects (Tables 3.2.1 and 3.2.2; Figure 3.2.1).

## Developmental Assessment and Follow-Up at Six Years of Age

Since one of the aims of any longitudinal study is to see the developmental pattern of any aspect over a period, it required the comparison of children at two different consecutive levels. In the present study, it was between children aged four and six years. The CD scores of all the

**Table 3.2.1:**
*Mean IQ and CD score of 4 years old cohort subjects*

| | CIE Scale of Intelligence | | | CD Test | | |
|---|---|---|---|---|---|---|
| | *No.* | *Mean IQ* | *SD* | *No.* | *Mean CD Score* | *SD* |
| **School Going Status** | | | | | | |
| School Going | 335 | 107.79 | 10.54 | 314 | 72.38 | 11.53 |
| Non-school Going | 547 | 94.34 | 11.5 | 237 | 59.24 | 12.41 |
| **Total** | **882** | **99.45** | **12.9** | **557** | **66.73** | **13.57** |
| **Education of Mother** | | | | | | |
| Illiterate/Semi-literate | 218 | 92.63 | 12.71 | 111 | 58.33 | 12.56 |
| Primary/Middle | 280 | 97.88 | 11.59 | 168 | 64.58 | 13.28 |
| Matric/High School | 205 | 103.81 | 11.83 | 140 | 72.07 | 11.76 |
| College | 98 | 108.41 | 11.56 | 68 | 74.5 | 10.47 |
| Not Known | 81 | 101.33 | 11.16 | 64 | 66.99 | 18.33 |
| **Per Capita Income (in ₹)** | | | | | | |
| ≤50. | 363 | 95.76 | 13.22 | 205 | 62.65 | 13.16 |
| 51–100 | 260 | 99.46 | 11.61 | 160 | 66.7 | 13.62 |
| 101–150 | 86 | 104.74*** | 13.41 | 57 | 70.97 | 13.33 |
| 151–200 | 41 | 105.58*** | 10.44 | 33 | 74 | 8.71 |
| 201+ | 51 | 108.82*** | 10.43 | 32 | 77.41 | 9.91 |
| Not Known | 81 | 101.33 | 11.16 | 64 | 66.99 | 13.33 |
| **Mother Employed Outside Home** | | | | | | |
| Yes | 65 | 104.29 | 12.69 | 40 | 69.64 | 14.19 |
| No | 780 | 99.24 | 12.8 | 487 | 66.64 | 13.32 |
| Not Known | 37 | 95.38 | 13.6 | 24 | 63.67 | 16.79 |
| **Total** | **882** | **99.45** | **12.9** | **551** | **66.73** | **13.57** |
| **No. of Siblings** | | | | | | |
| 1 | 213 | 101.6 | 13.11 | 32 | 72.53 | 13.07 |
| 2 | 177 | 98.7 | 12.98 | 149 | 71.19 | 12.81 |
| 3 | 127 | 98.08 | 12.37 | 160 | 67.38 | 12.64 |
| 4 | 69 | 94.08 | 14.89 | 92 | 65.31 | 12.44 |
| 5 | 33 | 95.07 | 10.12 | 57 | 61.52 | 14.77 |
| 6+ | 63 | 96.16 | 14.24 | 61 | 58.09 | 12.64 |
| **Total** | **882** | | | **551** | | |

(Table 3.2.1 *continued*)

(Table 3.2.1 *continued*)

| | CIE Scale of Intelligence | | | CD Test | | |
|---|---|---|---|---|---|---|
| | *No.* | *Mean IQ* | *SD* | *No.* | *Mean CD Score* | *SD* |
| **Type of Family** | | | | | | |
| Nuclear | 497 | 97.83 | 13.15 | 297 | 65.26 | 13.94 |
| Joint | 303 | 101.57 | 12.63 | 189 | 68.87 | 12.79 |
| Not Known | 82 | 101.42 | 11.11 | 65 | 67.23 | 13.36 |
| **Total** | **882** | **99.45** | **12.9** | **551** | **66.73** | **13.57** |
| **Number of Rooms** | | | | | | |
| Room is every thing | 143 | 93.93 | 12.9 | 83 | 60.72 | 12.03 |
| 1 | 306 | 97.13 | 12.33 | 180 | 64.8 | 13.89 |
| 2 | 260 | 102.76 | 12.9 | 161 | 70.08 | 13.27 |
| 3 | 54 | 105.94 | 11.77 | 38 | 70.82 | 12.18 |
| 4+ | 38 | 102.95 | 11.13 | 25 | 72.14 | 10.82 |
| Not Known | 81 | 101.33 | 11.16 | 64 | 66.99 | 13.33 |
| **Total** | **882** | **99.45** | **12.9** | **551** | **66.73** | **13.57** |

(1 vs 4+) sig at 5.0% level for CD test, (1 vs 4+) sig at 0.1% level for CIE scale.

| **Birth Order** | | | | | | |
|---|---|---|---|---|---|---|
| 1 | 151 | 112.48 | 11.18 | 91 | 70.23 | 11.96 |
| 2 | 178 | 101.93 | 13.74 | 98 | 67.66 | 13.83 |
| 3 | 144 | 99.18 | 13.22 | 92 | 65.42 | 13.19 |
| 4 | 116 | 98.3 | 12.51 | 57 | 65.74 | 12.59 |
| 5+ | 143 | 94.98 | 14.23 | 67 | 57.99 | 13.78 |
| Not Known | 150 | 98.86 | 10.83 | 146 | 69.15 | 13.18 |
| **Total** | **882** | **99.45** | **12.9** | **551** | **66.73** | **13.57** |

*5+ vs. 1, 2, 3 and 4 sig at 0.1% in CD test*

*5+ vs. 4 sig at 5.0% in CIE scale*

*5+ vs. 3 sig at 1.0% in CIE scale*

*5+ vs. 1, 2 sig at 0.1% in CIE scale*

| **Gender** | | | | | | |
|---|---|---|---|---|---|---|
| Male | 453 | 99.76 | 12.47 | 277 | 67.33 | 13.25 |
| Female | 428 | 99.13 | 13.39 | 271 | 66.13 | 13.81 |
| Not Known | 1 | 91.66 | – | 3 | 65.49 | 23.95 |
| **Total** | **882** | **99.45** | **12.9** | **551** | **66.73** | **13.57** |

No significant difference found

| | CIE Scale of Intelligence | | | CD Test | | |
|---|---|---|---|---|---|---|
| | No. | Mean IQ | SD | No | Mean CD Score | SD |
| **Education of Father** | | | | | | |
| Illiterate/Semi-literate | _ | _ | _ | 21 | 54.46 | 10.21 |
| Primary/Middle | _ | _ | _ | 145 | 60.76 | 13.51 |
| Matric/High School | _ | _ | _ | 211 | 67.94 | 12.75 |
| College | _ | _ | _ | 140 | 70.85 | 12.43 |
| Postgraduate | _ | _ | _ | 28 | 73.87 | 9.96 |
| Not Known | _ | _ | _ | 6 | 81.16 | 12.58 |
| **Total** | _ | _ | _ | **551** | **66.73** | **13.57** |

*Source:* Author.

*Notes:* *** Level of Significance for CIE Scale
1 vs. 2, 3, 4, and 5 significance at 0.1% level.
2 vs. 3, 4, and 5 significance at 0.1 % level.
Level of Significance for CD Test.
1 vs. 2 significance at 5.0% level; 1 vs. 3, 4 and 5 significance at 0.1%.
2 vs. 3 significance at 5.0%;2 vs. 4 significance at 1.0%.
2 vs. 5 significance at 0.1%;3 vs. 5 significance at 5%.

**Table 3.2.2:**
*CD scores of 6 years old cohort subjects*

| | CD Test | | |
|---|---|---|---|
| | No | Mean CD Score | SD |
| **School Going Status** | | | |
| School Going | 753 | 58.2 | 15.16 |
| Non-school Going | 18 | 37.2 | 12.86 |
| **Total** | **771** | **57.74** | **15.43** |
| **Education of Mother*** | | | |
| Illiterate/Semi-literate | 168 | 31.63*** | 14.4 |
| Primary/Middle | 247 | 54.81*** | 13.46 |
| Matric/High School | 178 | 63.64*** | 13.4 |
| College | 96 | 71.30*** | 11.91 |
| Not Known | 82 | 59.82 | 14.13 |

(Table 3.2.2 *continued*)

(Table 3.2.2 *continued*)

| | CD Test | | |
| | No | Mean CD Score | SD |
| --- | --- | --- | --- |
| **Per Capita Income (in ₹)** | | | |
| ≤50 | 294 | 50.84 | 14.43 |
| 51–100 | 226 | 58.11 | 14.12 |
| 101–150 | 77 | 63.91 | 14.55 |
| 151–200 | 43 | 68.11 | 10.89 |
| 201+ | 50 | 74.28 | 9.67 |
| Not Known | 81 | 59.98 | 14.17 |
| **Mother Employed Outside Home** | | | |
| Yes | 64 | 65.33 | 16.07 |
| No | 678 | 57.03 | 14.14 |
| Not Known | 29 | 57.02 | 16.5 |
| **Total** | **771** | **57.74** | **15.43** |
| **No. of Siblings** | | | |
| 1 | 16 | 70.96 | 12.05 |
| 2 | 159 | 66.77 | 12.22 |
| 3 | 212 | 61.46 | 14.14 |
| 4 | 174 | 53.85 | 14.8 |
| 5 | 91 | 51.01 | 14.7 |
| 6+ | 115 | 47.85 | 13.23 |
| **Total** | **771** | | |
| **Type of Family** | | | |
| Nuclear | 402 | 55.71 | 15.67 |
| Joint | 287 | 59.91 | 15.11 |
| Not Known | 82 | 59.87 | 14.97 |
| **Total** | **771** | **57.74** | **15.43** |
| Nuclear vs. Joint sig at 0.1% level | | | |
| **Number of Rooms** | | | |
| Room including kitchen | 112 | 49.83 | 13.76 |
| 1 | 247 | 54.64 | 15.87 |
| 2 | 239 | 61.13 | 14.46 |
| 3 | 54 | 62.58 | 12.83 |
| 4+ | 38 | 67.96 | 12.85 |
| Not Known | 81 | 59.96 | 14.17 |
| **Total** | **771** | **57.74** | **15.43** |

| | | CD Test | |
|---|---|---|---|
| | *No* | Mean CD *Score* | *SD* |
| **Birth Order** | | | |
| 1 | 119 | 61.93 | 14.81 |
| 2 | 164 | 60.87 | 14.26 |
| 3 | 130 | 57.11 | 15.13 |
| 4 | 78 | 54.08 | 13.82 |
| 5+ | 115 | 47.69 | 14.6 |
| Not Known | 165 | 60.74 | 15.22 |
| **Total** | **771** | **57.74** | **15.43** |
| **Education of Father** | | | |
| Illiterate/Semi-literate | 47 | 41.71 | 12.84 |
| Primary/Middle | 180 | 50.23 | 14.18 |
| Matric/High School | 305 | 57.28 | 13.56 |
| College | 187 | 66.86 | 12.52 |
| Postgraduate | 45 | 70.18 | 12.93 |
| Not Known | 6 | 52.32 | 20.24 |
| **Total** | **771** | **57.74** | **15.43** |

*Source:* Author.
*Notes:* *Education of mother statistical significance.
1 vs. 2, 3, and 4.
2 vs. 3 and 4; Significant at 0.1% level ***.

six-year-old children had gone down in comparison to the scores of four-year-old, giving a general impression that at the age of six either they had become relatively less intelligent or there was something different with the test itself, which caused such an effect.

This was not the first instance of such results being obtained. Most of the present tests have been devised on the theory of a constant general intelligence and, therefore, have failed to register adequately the developmental changes taking place on the constancy of mental scores over the childhood years for representative groups of children [68].

Moreover, the tests used were independent measures of cognitive abilities (unlike other age scales where, on the same test, different age groups are assessed in reference to age norms). The trends of the results of the six-year-old, which have emerged are closely akin to those of four years and are in agreement with hypothesis initially formulated.

**Figure 3.2.1:**
*CD scores in school going and not school going children at 6 years*

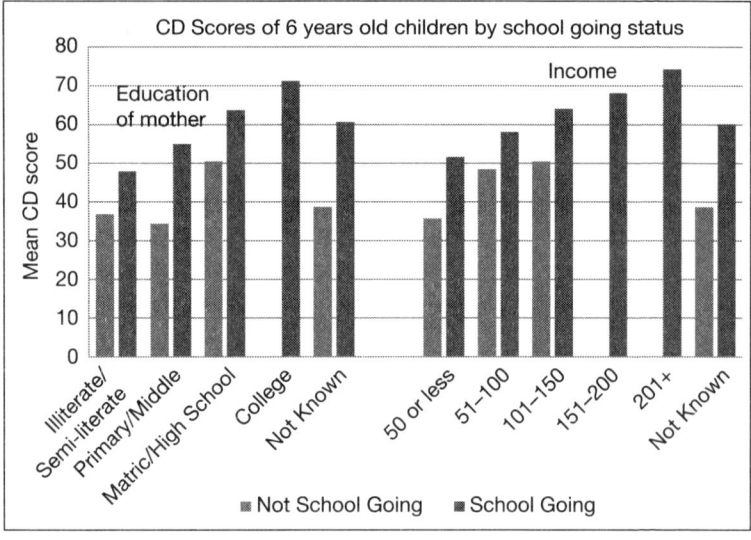

*Source:* Author.

# 3

# Nutrition

## Introduction

Nutrition in childhood, whether in health or disease, has always remained a major concern and a thrust area in national and international health policies. If a child is underfed or overfed or fed with an inappropriate kind of food, it has the potential to result in malnutrition and its related consequences in immediate or adult life.

In the late 1960s and the early 1970s, when this study was planned, the knowledge, appropriate investigative facilities, trained personnel, and data collection, monitoring, and analysis was limited. In view of this, our experience, and available resources, it was decided to assess the nutrition through physical growth monitoring and clinical observations. At this time, malnutrition was largely reflected as undernutrition. It occurred in the form of deficient calories, deficient proteins, or a combination of both. These clinically manifested as underweight, short stature, wasting, and micronutrient deficiencies and were the most commonly observed disorders. Overweight and obesity were hardly seen.

The initial objectives of this study were to find the prevalence of undernutrition by recording serial body growth measurement such as weight, length/height, head circumference, and mid-arm circumference at specified ages in childhood. As these were available in adult life, the objectives were revised to establish association between childhood body growth and BMI with chronic adult diseases. It also offered an opportunity to confirm Barker's hypothesis in Indian subjects from a low and middle-income country.

This part of the book will describe the nutritional status and occurrence of malnutrition at its both ends of undernutrition like stunting and overnutrition like obesity, and its causes and consequences. The body growth and composition will be described later in the chapter on adults on body growth and the development of chronic disease such as diabetes, hypertension, metabolic syndrome, and so forth.

## Malnutrition in Under Five Children

For nutrition and nutrition related problems, we focussed our attention in children up to 5 years of age as they are the most vulnerable group for survival and morbidity. Nutrition disorders are one of the most common disorders in childhood. The story of malnutrition may well begin in the intrauterine period when the foetus either fails to grow or the pregnancy terminates by early onset of labour resulting in preterm births, or it may grow at a faster rate due to maternal or foetal conditions. In the first instance, the infants are born with LBW; in the later, a preterm infant with LBW but the foetus grows at a faster rate than the infant born as a LGA infant.

The most common form of malnutrition is undernutrition in the developing world like in India. With the nutritional transition in last few decades, and with rapid lifestyle changes in food habits, the country is beginning to face the problem of overweight and obesity. It may begin any time during childhood from preschool period to adolescence.

The design of the study was to measure children at specific age periods every 6 months after 1 year of age for selective body measurements. No other regular clinical follow-up was done.

## Nutritional Assessment

Currently, several methods are used for the assessment of nutrition. These include anthropometry, biochemical, clinical examination, and dietary assessment by nutrition survey through a questionnaire. We used anthropometry and clinical examination by a medical officer to evaluate the nutritional profile. Several anthropometric measurements were serially recorded from birth at the specified age period till adult age. The measurements included body weight, length/height, head circumference, sitting height, and upper mid-arm circumference (UMAC). The details of the techniques of measurements are described elsewhere.

In order to evaluate the nutrition of the children, the WHO standard based on height, weight, and BMI for age and gender were used. The height, weight, and BMI of the individual children were converted to WHO height for age, weight for age, and BMI for age Z scores respectively. Based on the WHO criteria, they were classified as normal or stunted (short) using height for age Z score; wasted (thin) or overweight or obese using BMI for age WHO Z score or WHO Z scores for weight-for-height [67]. The criteria are:

## Undernutrition

### Stunted

WHO (Z score) height for age: $< -2.00$ Moderate Stunted

### Wasting

WHO (Z score) Weight for height $< -2$ Moderate
WHO (Z score) Weight for height $< -3$ Severe

### Overnutrition/Overweight/Obesity

WHO BMI for age Z score $< -2.00$ Thin
WHO BMI for age Z score $< -3.00$ Very thin
WHO BMI for age Z score $>+1.00$ Overweight
WHO BMI for age Z score $>+2.00$ Obese

## Undernutrition

Undernutrtion was commonly seen in the first 5 years of age. Overnutrition was also seen, but this was negligible and in less than 10%. Undernutrition was seen in all the three forms of underweight, wasting, and stunting from birth to 5 years (Table 3.3.1).

## Underweight

The underweight varied between 18 and 31% from birth to 5 years in the children. It was about 18–19% at birth and increased to about 30% at 2 years of age. It remained between 18.9 and 30.6% thereafter. The undernutriton increased significantly from 2 years and remained so till 5 years. The severe form of underweight was seen between 3.7% and 8.9% from birth to 5 years of age. It was maximum at 2 years with 8.9% occurrence (Table 3.3.1).

**Table 3.3.1:**
*Distribution by Z<−2 in the cohort subjects by gender at different ages for stunting, underweight, and wasting*

| Age in Months | Male N | Male % | Female N | Female % | P Value* |
|---|---|---|---|---|---|
| | | *Stunting* | | | |
| Birth | 3,444 | 12.9 | 3,194 | 10.8 | 0.011 |
| 6 | 3,572 | 21.3 | 3,285 | 16.6 | <0.001 |
| 12 | 2,787 | 35.3 | 2,569 | 32.3 | 0.019 |
| 24 | 2,794 | 46.7 | 2,544 | 45.7 | 0.475 |
| 36 | 2,673 | 46.8 | 2,443 | 51.0 | 0.003 |
| 48 | 2,499 | 41.8 | 2,327 | 48.5 | <0.001 |
| 60 | 2,205 | 36.2 | 2,085 | 41.9 | <0.001 |
| | | *Underweight* | | | |
| Birth | 3,586 | 18.9 | 3,221 | 18.3 | 0.493 |
| 6 | 3,576 | 24.2 | 3,292 | 23.6 | 0.591 |
| 12 | 2,790 | 25.1 | 2,573 | 23.0 | 0.073 |
| 24 | 2,774 | 30.9 | 2,528 | 29.9 | 0.420 |
| 36 | 2,655 | 25.1 | 2,434 | 30.6 | <0.001 |
| 48 | 2,489 | 19.9 | 2,317 | 27.8 | <0.001 |
| 60 | 2,212 | 18.9 | 2,086 | 26.4 | <0.001 |
| | | *Wasting* | | | |
| Birth | 3,247 | 17.8 | 2,947 | 18.5 | 0.531 |
| 6 | 3,569 | 12.5 | 3,286 | 12.6 | 0.913 |
| 12 | 2,783 | 11.1 | 2,566 | 9.6 | 0.073 |
| 24 | 2,770 | 10.5 | 2,520 | 7.7 | <0.001 |
| 36 | 2,652 | 5.0 | 2,432 | 4.7 | 0.696 |
| 48 | 2,485 | 3.0 | 2,313 | 3.7 | 0.171 |
| 60 | 2,204 | 3.1 | 2,081 | 3.1 | 1.000 |

*Source:* Author.
*Note:* * P value represents gender difference.

## Wasting

Wasting was seen to be more prevalent in the first 2 years than in 3–5 years of age. It varied from 10–12% from 0–2 years as compared to 3–5% in later years. It occurred to be maximum at birth and was significantly higher in females at 2 years of age. The severe form of wasting was seen to be most common at birth with 5.0%. It was seen as an uncommon problem with prevalence of about 1% in less than 2 years (Table 3.3.1).

## Stunting

Stunting was the most striking problem of undernutrition. It was seen in almost 50% of the children at 2 to 3 years of age and varied between 35 and 51% between 2 and 5 years. The prevalence of stunting was significantly higher in males as compared to females throughout the first five years, except at 2 years of age when it was almost the same in both males and females. The severe form of stunting varied from 11.2% to 19.0% from 1–5 years of age. It appears to be most frequent in 18.19% at 2–3 years of age and remained so in 10% of cases at 5 years of age (Table 3.3.1).

The children appeared to be most vulnerable at 2–3 years of age. The female children seemed to be more significantly affected than the males. The result supports the general observations that nutrition in the first 5 years is extremely important. It is critical in the first 2 years.

A comparison between boys and girls revealed an interesting pattern. The prevalence of wasting significantly increased in the third, fourth, and fifth year of life in girls as compared to boys. But the underweight prevalence was similar for boys and girls. Stunting followed a pattern similar to wasting, and the prevalence increased in the girls as compared to boys from 3 years. These findings are of interest as it may be due to discrimination between a boy and a girl in the family. Alternately, it could be that the girls begin to follow their normal growth pattern.

The cohort data collected prospectively suggest a significant number of the children to be born underweight, wasted, and stunted from birth, with its occurrence increasing to maximum at 2–3 years of age. The size of an infant born at birth was thus either small due to foetal growth retardation, or preterm birth, or a combination of both. The prevalence of wasting, undernutrition, and stunting recorded at birth showed a significant

**Table 3.3.2:**
*Prevalence of severe malnutrition Z score SD≤3 in the cohort subjects at different ages for stunting, underweight, and wasting*

| Age (in Months) | N | Severe Stunting (<–3 SD)% | N | Severe Underweight (<–3 SD)% | N | Severe Wasting (<–3 SD)% |
|---|---|---|---|---|---|---|
| Birth | 6,638 | 3.1 | 6,807 | 4.5 | 6,194 | 5.1 |
| 6 | 6,857 | 4.7 | 6,868 | 7.6 | 6,855 | 3.3 |
| 12 | 5,356 | 11.2 | 5,363 | 7.6 | 5,349 | 2.3 |
| 24 | 5,338 | 18.1 | 5,302 | 8.9 | 5,290 | 1.1 |
| 36 | 5,116 | 19.0 | 5,089 | 6.8 | 5,084 | 0.5 |
| 48 | 4,826 | 14.8 | 4,806 | 4.7 | 4,798 | 0.3 |
| 60 | 4,290 | 10.2 | 4,298 | 3.7 | 4,285 | 0.2 |

*Source:* Author.

increase, especially in stunting at 2 years of age. The severe form was also seen in all the three forms of undernutrition from birth to 5 years of age (Table 3.3.2, Figure 3.3.1). Severe stunting was seen in 10%–19% of the children. Stunting is regarded as an outcome of foetal growth retardation, feeding practices including disregard for the recommendation of exclusive breastfeeding till 6 months of age, early and inadequate complementary nutritional feeding, poor immunization compliance, and exposure to recurrent infections. The study demonstrates the relevance of considering the first 1,000 days, including the intrauterine period, as perhaps the most critical and precious years in the lives of human beings.

The causes contributing to the problem of undernutrition varied from environment to maternal health and education and socio-economic factors. These included type of family, sanitation, housing, maternal education, per capita income, maternal age, parity, LBW, and prematurity, All these factors were highly significant.

## Head Circumference

The smaller head circumference or head size was seen in 7.3% of children at birth, 10.3% at 2 years, and 6.1% at 5 years. The head size is a reflection of brain growth. It remained small and did not show any catch up growth. No apparent cause except being a small child was observed (Table 3.3.3).

**Figure 3.3.1:**
*Prevalence of stunting, underweight, and wasting at different age in cohort subjects*

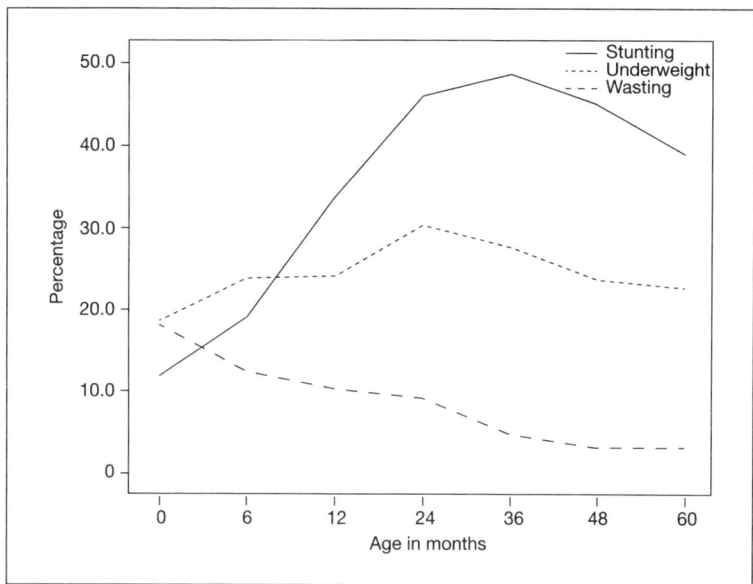

*Source:* Author.

**Table 3.3.3:**
*Distribution for WHO head circumference at different age for Z score < −2 in cohort subjects*

| Age (in Months) | N | WHO Head Circumference for Age Z Score < −2% |
|---|---|---|
| Birth | 6,605 | 7.3 |
| 6 | 6,830 | 13.6 |
| 12 | 5,326 | 12.0 |
| 24 | 5,309 | 10.3 |
| 36 | 5,101 | 9.0 |
| 48 | 4,781 | 7.8 |
| 60 | 4,189 | 6.1 |

*Source:* Author.

## Age Independent Measurements of Undernutrition

### Upper Mid-arm Circumference

The UMAC measurement is considered an independent measure of nutrition. Undernutrition is diagnosed if the UMAC is <11.5 cm. It was 19.5% between the ages of 18 and 30 months and decreased to 9.7% at five years of age. It also confirmed the decline in undernutrition prevalence with increasing age (Table 3.3.4).

These measurements were available in children between 24 and 72 months. UMAC had an excellent correlation with weight in children of either sex between 24 and 78 months. Thereafter, though a high correlation was observed in girls, the boys had a lower UMAC correlation to weight. No possible reason could be assigned to such a variation through the present data. However, review of published data reveals that UMAC to weight correlation in children under 5 years has been variable.

Shakir [68] had suggested an UMAC of 13.5 cm as being useful in screening for malnutrition. Table 3.3.4 provides the distribution of cases with the mid-upper-arm circumference (MUAC) observed in this study. Using this cut-off value, it was observed in the present study that an UMAC of 13.5 cm had a low sensitivity and high specificity in detecting malnutrition. These findings were consistent with other reports.

**Table 3.3.4:**
*Distribution for WHO MUAC for age Z score <−2 and MUAC <11.5 in different age groups of cohort subjects (UMAC measurement is available only after 1.8 years of age)*

| Age Groups (in years) | N | WHO MUAC for Age Z Score <−2% | MUAC <11.5 cm*% |
|---|---|---|---|
| 1.8–3.0 | 1,140 | 19.5 | 1.0 |
| 3.0–3.5 | 1,550 | 13.5 | 0.5 |
| 3.5–4.0 | 1,928 | 12.8 | 0.1 |
| 4.0–4.5 | 2,222 | 9.7 | 0.0 |
| 4.5–5.0 | 3,410 | 9.7 | 0.1 |

*Source:* Author.

**Note:** *Current definition for severe acute malnutrition in children aged 6 months to 5 years.

# PART 4

# Transition to Adult Phase

# 1

# Assembling the Cohort

In 1991 the NDBC successfully completed its foundation to child-hood phase. It was largely due to the commitment of the NDBC team (Figure 4.1.1) and cohorts cooperation.

The NDBC project was closed in 1991 after completion of the child-hood and adolescent phase. However, it's data files, records, original cards, and protocols were all destroyed due to an accidental fire and data files stored in magnetic tapes ASCII coded format in 2,400 ft (feet) spoolers were misplaced. The data manager had left no code books or details of the data storage of different files in the spooler's tapes. The writer had only kept some printed data sheets and files for personal historical records.

**Figure 4.1.1:**
*The NDBC research group*

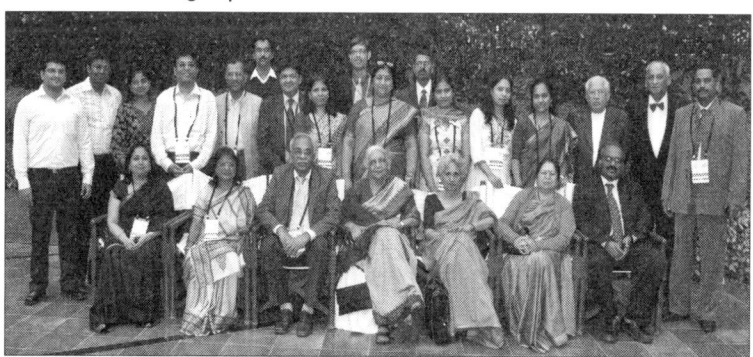

*Source:* Author.

## Assembling the Cohort

In 1994, at the time of the VIII Asian Congress of Paediatrics at Hotel Ashok, New Delhi, I met Professor David Barker and discussed the feasibility to test Barker's hypothesis of foetal origin of adult disease in the NDBC. Subsequently, Professor Bhargava and Professor H. P. S. Sachdev attended a Society for Nutrition Education and Health Action (SNEHA) workshop organized by Professor Anand Pandit at Khandala in August 1994 and had a meeting with Professor David Barker and Dr Caroline Fall to discuss the possibility of further follow-up of the NDBC. It was then decided to revive the NDBC project and a preliminary survey was planned to re-establish contact with the cohorts with a financial grant from MRC, Southampton, United Kingdom (UK).

The magnetic tapes in which the addresses of the cohorts were recorded were misplaced and not available. Hence, a list of cohorts was prepared from an old register which was used to maintain records of addresses when posting official letters under certificate of posting to cohorts. The last posting to cohorts was made in 1985. Letters were sent to over 3,000 cohort families regarding the intended visit of the project team to re-establish the contact and update certain information. In the meantime, an advertisement was made for recruitment of the staff in a leading newspaper. A pro forma for updating personal and family details, addresses, and contact details was developed and pretested in the field. It was then translated into Hindi language to facilitate accurate collection of information by the lay interviewers.

The response to the advertisement was very poor and hence direct recruitment of limited staff was done. The field interviewers were trained in pro forma administration and data collection. Fortunately, we could employ some former staff who had earlier worked in the project and were familiar with the study area, addresses, and families of the cohort.

### Tracing the Cohorts

The follow-up for retracing was broadly divided into an inner or the original Lajpat Nagar-IV project area and an outer area of Delhi where some cohorts had shifted their residence from the original area. The actual follow-up began in June 1995. This was slow as the field interviewers were totally untrained and unfamiliar with the nature of work.

The number of field interviewers that could be employed was fewer. In addition, the survey was done in the summer months during the vacation time of school children. The families did not like to be disturbed in the afternoon and many families were away from Delhi. The survey was planned as a house-to-house survey and personal contact with cohorts to minimize the loss to follow-up. The inner areas of the project were further divided into 10 sub-areas. A team of two interviewers visited each sub-area. The outer area was visited after completing the follow-up of the inner area. The visit to the cohort was categorized as available or as permanent or temporary loss. The completed questionnaires were returned to the supervisor who cross-checked each one of them and sent it for data entry. In case the cohort was not available to the field worker, then the cohort was revisited by the field supervisor to ensure that all efforts to contact them had been done. Only after a failed third attempt was the subject categorized as a permanent loss. In case of a refusal to provide the information, the supervisor or project consultant visited the family.

## Problems Encountered During Retracing

Several problems were encountered during the retracing of the follow-up. Contact was being initiated after a gap of several years. The staff was on a short-term appointment. The survey was conducted in the hottest months of summer. Then the rainy season began and the inclement weather made it even more difficult to complete the task. One of the major handicaps was lack of project transport as we found it difficult to find temporary short distance transport to commute to different parts of the area. The taxis or three-wheeler auto rickshaws did not want to wait till an enquiry or a conversation with the cohorts or informers could be completed. Many houses were found locked due to summer vacations. Several families had migrated to other parts of the city or left the area without leaving a forwarding address or information.

## Locating Data Tapes and Deciphering/Decoding Them

The data collection, its supervision during collection, review after collection of data, data entry, and its checks and balances were one of the highest priorities of the project. The project was very fortunate to always have outstanding, committed data managers and supervisors with bio-statistician and software programmers who managed enormous needs of the data including storage and its analysis for publication. They had to meet numerous challenges and difficulties of varying kinds and unforeseen circumstances and obstructions that came in the preservation, storage, and recovery of the data from the time when the capital city of India had only one computer centre and that too located in the Planning Commission of the Government of India. After the closure of the project in 1991, the data tapes were misplaced and were found with difficulty as junk in a store. There were no back up files, registers, or code books to indicate which tape stored what. We had found 29 data tapes but are still unaware if there were more tapes which we never recovered.

The data was stored in magnetic tapes in ASCII coded format tapes, 2,400 ft spoolers. These were created between 1970 and 1990. Most of the tapes are BASF/ENDURA (for use at 800 BPI through 6250 BPI) and created on IBM 360/44 machines as also on INTERDATA 8/32 machines.

Most of the tapes have been read and the data transferred, but 9 out of 29 tapes could not be converted. The perceived reason for this was that the tapes had not been stored in a proper manner. Some tapes were found after the exercise of converting the available tapes was over. Some tapes were labelled and blocked, which needed specific codes or tools and drives to run and read. However, our efforts to find a drive in the city and across India have now failed.

# 2

# The Beginning of the Adult Period

In 1998, we had the first of the many adult phase projects entitled 'Maternal Nutrition, Foetal Growth, and Coronary Risk Factors in Young Indian Adults: 1998–2002' sanctioned. This was a collaborative project between Professor Barker and colleagues from MRC Southampton, UK, and Professor Bhargava and colleagues in New Delhi with a grant from the British Heart Foundation, UK (Figure 4.2.1). The

**Figure 4.2.1:**
*The adult phase research group*

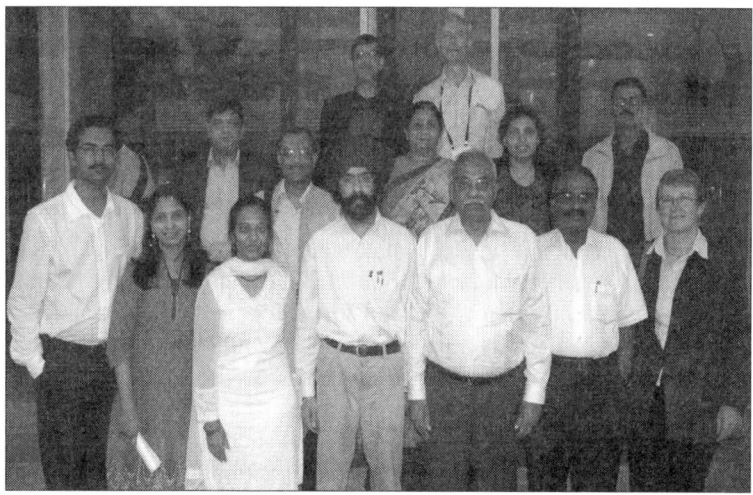

*Source:* Author.

objective was to investigate the association between birth weight, body growth, and body composition during childhood and chronic adult disease including impaired glucose tolerance (IGT), diabetes mellitus, lipid aberrations, and cardiovascular diseases.

The results of this project encouraged further work on these problems and the study was extended by another grant from British Heart Foundation in 2006–09 in collaboration with Professor Caroline Fall to investigate 'the changes in the endothelium of the blood vessels, pro-inflammatory and pro-thrombotic factors in predisposing and/or causation of atherosclerosis and CADs in adults.' It had also emerged from the NDBC data that growth in early life may predict adult bone health, and thus the study was enlarged to include the relationship of height and BMI during childhood with adult bone mineral content (BMC), bone density (aBMD and bone mineral apparent density [BMAD]), and estimated volumetric density.

In 2015, we have been sanctioned another grant in collaboration with Professor Fall from the British Heart Foundation in recognition of the earlier works and publications by the NDBC group on cardiovascular diseases with reference to birth weight related to gestational age, body growth, BMI, and myocardial abnormalities. This is to be related to current cardiometabolic risk factors and those measured 12–16 years ago in young adulthood, smoking and lower physical activity and its association with LBW for gestational age, lower weight in infancy, and faster BMI gain during late childhood. The current project too falls within the ambit of the original objectives of the NDBC, which is to pursue the story of LBW and its outcome.

Continuing the interest in LBW, Professor Bhargava met Professor Peter Gluckman from Auckland University, New Zealand, in a SNEHA annual meeting in Khandala in 2006. Professor Gluckman proposed a collaboration with the NDBC group to determine the 'economic cost of being born LBW during a life course'. The project was intended to develop an economic model, which could estimate this cost as such information was not available for developing countries. It was believed that this would be extremely useful for policy-makers and planners in countries where LBW is a national problem. Information so generated would be useful in determining the potential benefit of interventions in prevention rather than facing lifelong consequences of being born small.

In 2004, the NDBC research group found another direction in collaboration with four other leading similar cohorts from low middle-income countries of the world. These cohorts with their respective principal investigators included Professor L. Adair, The Cebu Longitudinal Health and Nutrition Survey (Philippines; CEBU-1963); Professor R. Martorell, The Institute of Central America and Panama Nutrition Trial (Guatemala; INCAP-1969); Professor L. Richter, The Birth to Twenty Study (South Africa; BT20-1990); Professor. C. Victora, Pelotas Birth Cohort Study (Brazil) 1982; and Professor Santosh Bhargava, the NDBC (Delhi; NDBC-1969), and the group is commonly known with its acronym as 'The COHORTS' [69].

The COHORTS group has a wide but common interest and investigated the influence of maternal and child undernutrition in early to mid- and late childhood and adolescence growth, birth weight, and gestational age on development of chronic adult diseases. More importantly, it studied the impact of these on human capital development, which included attainment of adult height, earning capacity and education, and, more importantly, the influence on the birth weight of the next generation of the offspring.

The 'COHORTS' group also focused its attention on early life period of first 2 years and showed that the maximal potential for gains in human capital development occur in this period. This pioneering work perhaps lead to the coining of the term the 'first 1,000 days', which includes the intrauterine period after conception and the first 2 years of life.

The other significant contribution of this collaboration has been to see the impact of exposure of exclusive breastfeeding in the first 6 months on the development of adult diseases such as hypertension, obesity, schooling, and CD. It investigated the influence in early life to environment, parent's education, and access to health facilities and others on body growth and composition. The COHORT group research efforts were supported by several grants from the Wellcome Trust UK from 2006 to 2012.

In 2012, the Bill and Melinda Gates Foundation found merit in supporting the COHORT group in its effort to further examine the influence of preterm birth, rapid growth before and after 2 years, stunting at 2 years, and poverty, parental education, and exclusive breastfeeding on adult health and development. The primary aim of the grant was to publish results of these five unique cohorts' data for global public health policies and concerns. In 2015, we have received another grant from this organization to investigate the 'Healthy Birth, Growth, and Development Knowledge Integration COHORTS team's Analysis Plan'. The objective is to determine the extent to which circumstances at birth (characterized by term/preterm status, birth weight, and mode of delivery) and postnatal growth patterns predict indicators of human capital development that are mediated through brain function (cognitive attainment and measures of schooling attainment) and early-adult employment in low and middle-income country settings.

Another investigation which has been in progress has been to develop an Indian model to estimate the health costs associated with type 2 diabetes in Indians in association with Stanford University, USA. The NDBC has closely followed occurrence of diabetes in its cohorts and has the necessary data to make such an effort.

The NDBC collaboration continues to grow and is now a part of a 52-investigator team from 17 counties across the globe on the 'economic impact of poverty related risk factors during the first 1,000 days for cognitive and human capital development'. The project aims to address four key poverty related risk factors during the first 1,000 days. These are malnutrition, infection, poor management of pregnancy and birth complication and lack of cognitive stimulation and nurturing, and calculating the cost of selected related intervention over the life. The team 1,000+ proposes an innovative strategy to improve the understanding. This is being pursued with a grant from Grand Challenges Canada (GCC) in 2014.

The richness of the information prompted us to investigate the genetic influences on body growth, rate of body growth, and body composition. The project is investigating association of genes with metabolic perturbations including diabetes (carbohydrates), dyslipidaemia (fats), and excess body growth (overweight). These genetic investigations focused on association of genetic variations with serial BMI changes from birth to adulthood and CAD factors. Another aspect of investigation was to study autoimmune markers of diabetes with birth weight, ponderal index (measure of thinness at birth), BMI, and BMI trajectories.

The genetic aspects continue to interest us, and hence the work was extended to study the generic determinants of birth weight and growth trajectories and influence of parental genotype on these growth parameters. Another dimension of LBW being investigated includes the determination of size at birth, infant and child growth on telomere length, and telomerase activity in childhood. The studies on genes and genetic aspects have been supported by the ICMR and the Department of Biotechnology of the Government of India.

The NDBC group has been proactively following research with national researchers and national institutions by active association and collaborative research. The national organizations, which have been supportive of our efforts, have been the ICMR, and the Department of Science and Technology and Department of Biotechnology of the Government of India. The national institutions which have collaborated with us have been the All India Institute of Medical Sciences, Public Health Foundation of India, Maulana Azad Medical College, Sitaram Bhartia Institute of Science and Research, Center for Chronic Diseases Control, S.L. Jain Hospital, The Heart Centre, Institute of Genomics and Integrative Biology, and others.

The NDBC has been very active in conducting intramural research with focus on the F2 generation are children of the NDBC. It has pursued several pilot projects on this generation including obesity, cardiovascular risk factors, behaviour problems, and hand grip strength. In an international collaborative study with Professor Sumit Bhargava from Stanford University, USA, it has studied several aspects on sleep problems in children, particularly the trans-generation effects in trios or the three generations of the cohort.

# 3

# Re-establishing the New Delhi Birth Cohort

## Reviving the New Delhi Birth Cohort

At the beginning of the adult phase of the NDBC, it was expected that 3,337 or 40.7% of the original cohort would be available for follow-up in this phase. In order to reach them and to establish contact with them, it was decided to first write a letter in English and Hindi to inform them about the intended visit. While it was being done, the team of field workers was being trained and briefed about the methodology for retracing and follow-up. The process involved a visit to the house personally to contact the cohort or his family member, obtain the telephone number and contact details, and arranging a suitable time to meet and to reach them. In the last 47 years, the cohorts have shifted residence in Delhi, gone to other parts and cities of India, and spread globally. It was largely marriage- and occupation-driven migration Hence, in case a subject was not located or found at the address, revisits were made and the neighbours and other persons in the locality were contacted to obtain their new addresses. Sometimes it needed repeated visits to locate the correct address.

## Current Status of the Cohort

The NDBC has traversed through exciting times in India in the last five decades. During this time India has undergone a complete transformation in both rural and urban regions and especially in the large metro cities like New Delhi. The city of New Delhi happens to be the capital of India and the capital of the state of Delhi. This pioneering work perhaps, lead to the coining of the term the 'First 1,000 days' which includes the intra-uterine period after conception and the first 2 years of life.

The other significant contribution of this collaboration has been to see the impact was known for government offices and government employees transformed to a cosmopolitan city with influx of population from different states of the country. This has turned the city from a city of governance to be a city with industrial houses and industries, business centres, large offices, changes in public and private transport mode and in housing from single houses to huge multi-storey large flat complexes, and so forth. All these changes have been influencing the NDBC lives in one way or another. These changes and its influence will be described later.

Technically, the NDBC has grown from a single generation of the F1 cohorts to four generations of the family cohort. The F0 is the first generation and they are the parents of the NDBC; the F1 generation is the NDBC, the F2 generation is the children of the cohorts, and the F3 is the generation of the grandchildren of the cohorts (Figure 4.3.1).

**Figure 4.3.1:**
*The four generations of the NDBC*

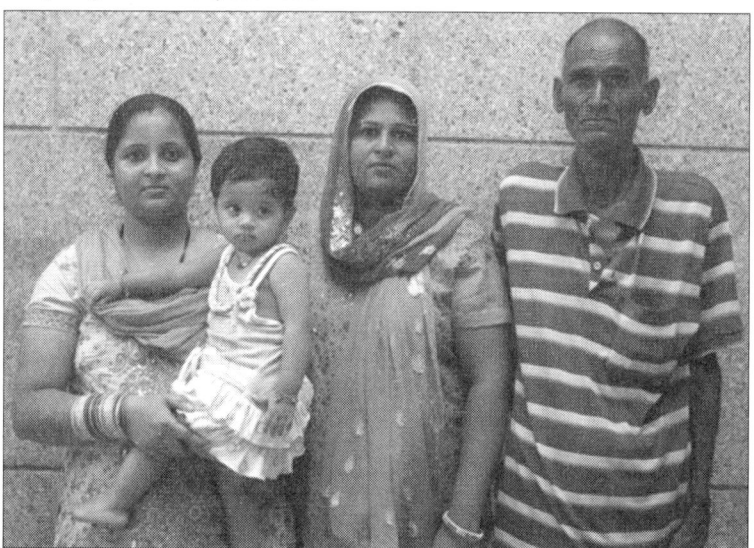

*Source:* Author.

In the foundation years of 1969–73, we had 8,181 cohorts (F1). Over the period of 47 years we have lost about 6,000 cohort due to several reasons including demolition of colonies with complete displacement and migration of cohort, moving out of the area without leaving an address, or refusal to cooperate or having expired. We have during the years 1969 to 2015 had eight different phases of the NDBC follow-up at different time periods and intervals. The last complete retracing follow-up of Phase VII was done between 2006 and 2009. We are currently in the Phase VIII of 2012–15 follow-up. The cohort follow-up in different phases is illustrated in Figure 4.3.2.

In Phase I, in between 1969 and 1973, we had 8,181 cohorts. In the Phase II of the cohort tracing round in 1975–80, we had 7,119 and in the Phase III of tracing round between 1984 and 1987, the cohort number dropped to 4,705. The final phase, Phase IV of the childhood to adolescence and reaching the adult age, was between 1988 and 1990 in which we had 3,337 cohort subjects, but due to constraints of the fund, the follow-up was limited to cohorts reaching the age of 17–20 years.

Thus, the preconception to conception and birth to childhood and to adult phases of the project which began from founding in 1969 were completed in 1991 and the project was officially closed.

We had the next phase (V) of tracing round in 1998–2003 to revive the contact with cohorts. At this time we had 3,337 cohorts, having lost 4,844 (59.2%) during the period 1969–2003. The next round of tracing was Phase VI from 2003 to 2006 when we registered 2,584 cohorts, losing an additional 753 (22.5%). In Phase VII of 2006–09, we lost further 825 (31.9%) cohorts, thus leaving 1,759 as the available cohort for follow-up. However, the numbers of cohorts which may be available during a follow-up are at times variable. This is due to cohorts being reported as lost and then by chance during an enquiry to be found again by some leads on new address. We are now in an ongoing Phase VIII in 2015 and from an original listing of 3,352 cohorts we have been now able to track 2,105 cohorts.

## Methodology of NDBC Studies in Different Periods of Adult Phase

### Organization of the Field Clinics

In contrast to the childhood phase, the follow-up method and assessment had to be altered in adulthood. In the childhood phase, it was entirely

**Figure 4.3.2:**
*Cohorts in different phases of study 1969–2015*

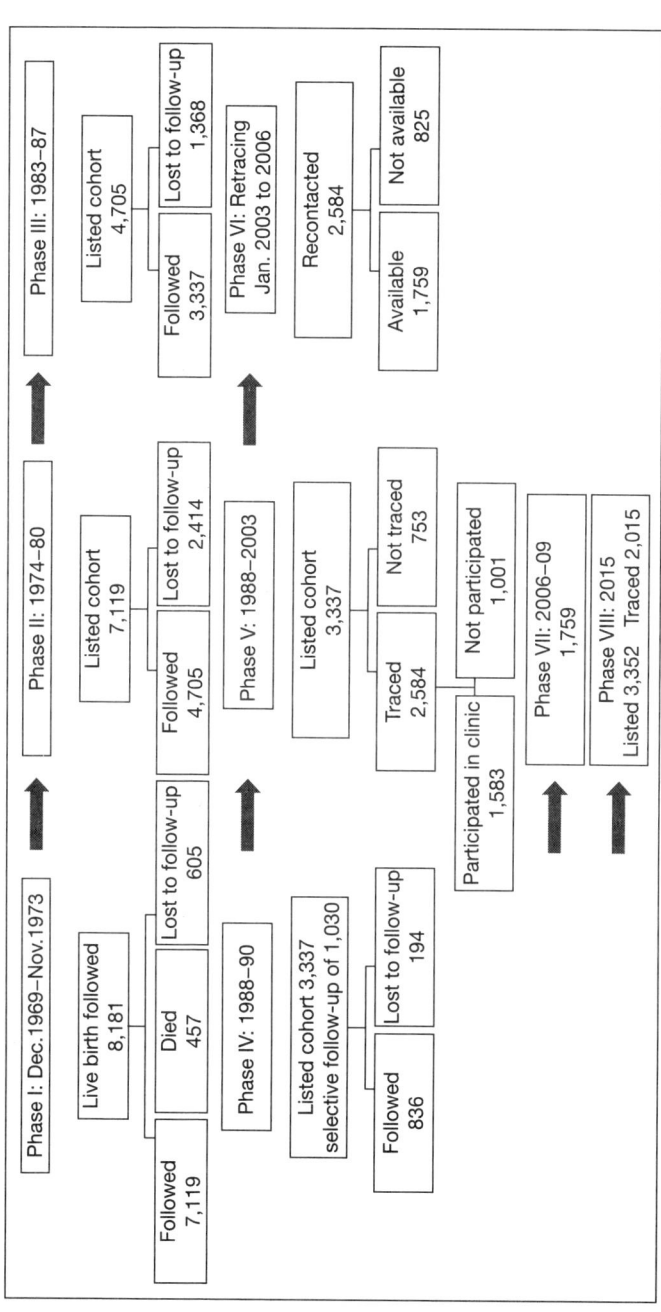

**Source:** Author.

a home-based follow-up but in the adult phase it had to be totally a field-based follow-up and assessment. The organization of a field clinic involved pre-clinic activity, the actual field clinic activity, and the post-clinic activity.

## Pre-clinic Activities

Pre-clinic activity involved identifying the specific area in the field, fixing a venue for the clinic, making a list of the cohorts to be invited to attend clinic from a central list, making a telephone call to the cohort for enquiring about availability on the clinic days and dates, and fixing the timing and venue of the field clinic. Thereafter, a staff made a visit to the home to provide written details of the clinic, reconfirming their appointment in the clinic and clarifying any doubts. Finally, 1–2 days prior to the clinic, another telephone reminder was given to the family and cohort.

## Clinic Activity

One day prior to the clinic, the venue had to be rented in the neighbourhood of those being invited to clinics for setting up the place for the next day clinic which starts in the early morning. The clinic venue could be a large hall or number of rooms in a building, usually on the same floor but sometimes on two different floors of a building. For the clinic, the place was divided into different sections for different activities. These included stations for registration, pro forma completion, medical examination, anthropometry rooms and separate enclosures for male and female subjects, blood collection and sampling, and so on.

The pre-clinic, clinic, and post-clinic activity is summarized in Figure 4.3.3.

In the clinic, the cohort is again explained the objectivities and purpose of clinic, and a written consent is obtained with the information sheet. After obtaining the written consent to participate in the study, the subjects rotate through the different sections of the clinic, which is divided by functions. These included completing different sets of pro formas of medical and clinical examination and anthropometric measurements including weight, height, waist and hip circumference, bio-impedance, hand grip strength, skin fold thickness, and blood sample collection for different biochemical and other tests (Figures 4.3.4). In the clinic, the cohorts were served refreshments after completion of the scheduled tests.

**Figure 4.3.3:**
*Pre-field clinic, clinic, and post-clinic activities*

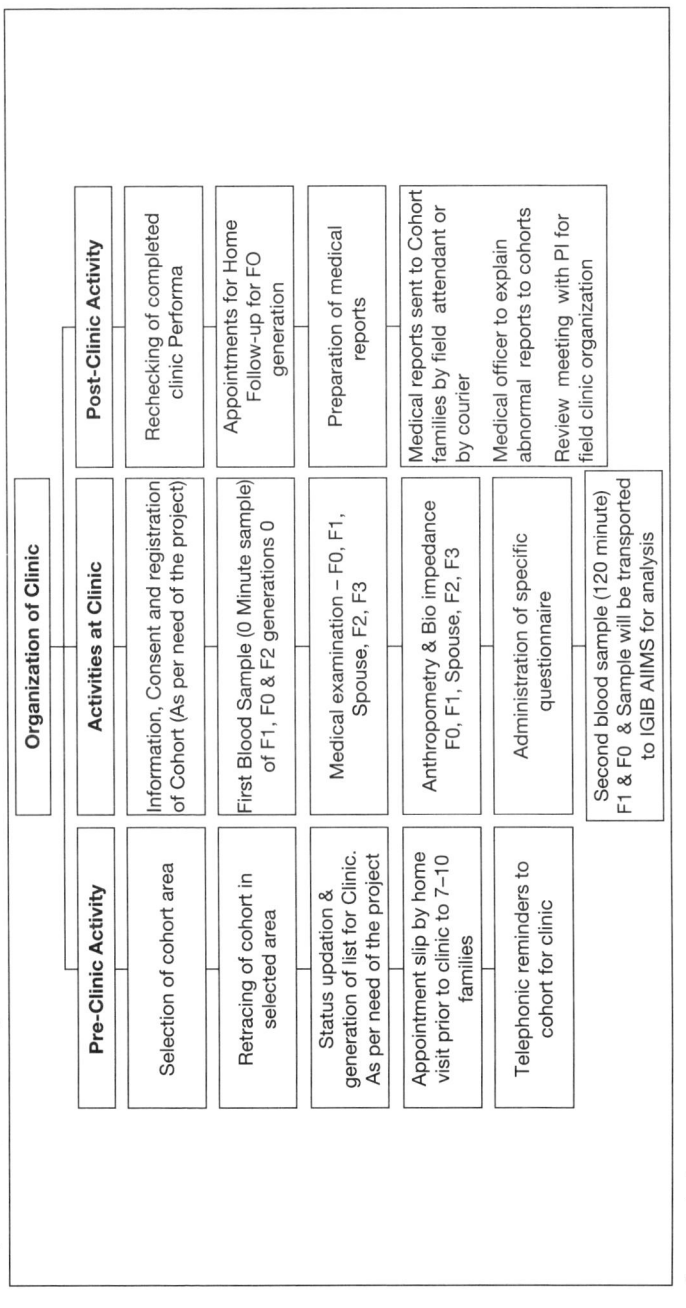

**Organization of Clinic**

| Pre-Clinic Activity | Activities at Clinic | Post-Clinic Activity |
|---|---|---|
| Selection of cohort area | Information, Consent and registration of Cohort (As per need of the project) | Rechecking of completed clinic Performa |
| Retracing of cohort in selected area | First Blood Sample (0 Minute sample) of F1, F0 & F2 generations 0 | Appointments for Home Follow-up for FO generation |
| Status updation & generation of list for Clinic. As per need of the project | Medical examination – F0, F1, Spouse, F2, F3 | Preparation of medical reports |
| Appointment slip by home visit prior to clinic to 7–10 families | Anthropometry & Bio impedance F0, F1, Spouse, F2, F3 | Medical reports sent to Cohort families by field attendant or by courier |
| Telephonic reminders to cohort for clinic | Administration of specific questionnaire | Medical officer to explain abnormal reports to cohorts |
| | Second blood sample (120 minute) F1 & F0 & Sample will be transported to IGIB AIIMS for analysis | Review meeting with PI for field clinic organization |

***Source:*** Author.

**Figure 4.3.4:**
*Schedules/pro formas used in the adult phase VI–VIII studies*

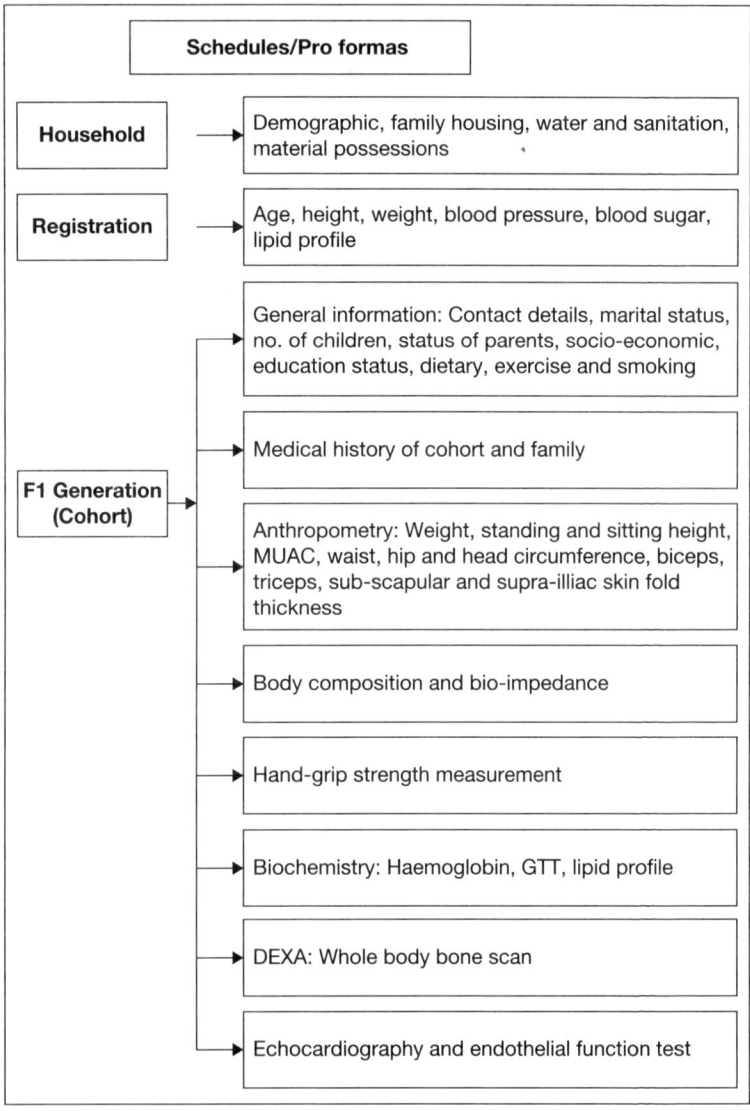

*Source:* Author.

## Post-clinic Activity

The post-clinic activity involved rechecking of the forms, their corrections, obtaining laboratory reports, and forwarding these for data entry to data manger. Once the data entry was finished, a complete report of the clinic is prepared and sent to the concerned individual, personally or by courier. If the reports are abnormal, these are explained by the NDBC medical officer and they are always advised to contact their physician.

The pre-clinic, clinic, and post-clinic activities for completion of all tasks takes nearly 3–4 weeks. The clinic are usually organized twice or thrice in a month on weekdays and holidays.

In case of a missed appointment, a visit is made to the cohort to enquire the reasons for missing the clinic and taking corrective action, if possible.

# 4

# Environments, Social and Cultural Changes

At the beginning of the 1998–2003 phase, we had tracked 2,583 cohorts. However, only 1,583 (61.2%) agreed to be interviewed for socio-cultural and other aspects. A detailed questionnaire-based survey was done to determine their socio-cultural and environmental characteristics, sanitation, water supply and living standards, wealth generation, food habits, physical activity pattern, and current health problems. This was done with a view to see the changes during the last 25–30 years when the cohorts were born and when they had become young adults between 26 and 29 years of age. This also offered an opportunity to record observations on the secular trends with a generation change in the same families living in the same surroundings.

1.  **Cohort Characteristics**
    Amongst the 1,583 subjects, males significantly dominated with 899 (56.8%); 75% of the cohort population were married, 24.0% were unmarried, and a few who widowed or divorced. The presence of divorce was a social change as hardly any divorces were recorded in the 1969–73 phase.

    The family pattern remained unchanged as most of them were nuclear families. The families looked more prosperous. The socio-economic status had improved considerably. Those with an income of ₹ 50–200 per month moved into an apparently larger bracket of income. It was difficult to ask their actual income due to fear of tax regulations. The self-owned houses were given on rent. Many of cohorts had started their own additional business in addition to their regular jobs or had become independent entrepreneurs. The cohorts were better educated than their parents and had several additional different kinds of professions than their parents.

2. **Housing, Sanitation, and Water Supply**
   Over 99% lived in flats or independent *pucca* houses with very few in *jhuggies* (slums) as compared to their parents. This too was a very noticeable stark change. Almost 90% had tap water for drinking and 10% used bore or tube well water. No hand pump or other source of water was used for drinking. This period of 1998–2002 was vastly different then earlier phase of 1969–73 (Figure 4.4.1).

3. **Education**
   The educational status had also undergone a significant change. The cohorts had received much better education than their parents. There were hardly any illiterates, as compared to almost 10% in their parents. The number of cohorts who received education from primary to high school decreased to 41.3% as compared to 49.4% in their parents. In contrast, the number of graduates in cohorts had increased from 18.3% in their parent's time to 43.9%. Similarly, the number of postgraduates had also increased from 8.1% in parents to 13.3% in their cohort children (Figure 4.4.2).

**Figure 4.4.1:**
*Distribution for water and sanitation facilities for F1 cohort in adult phase*

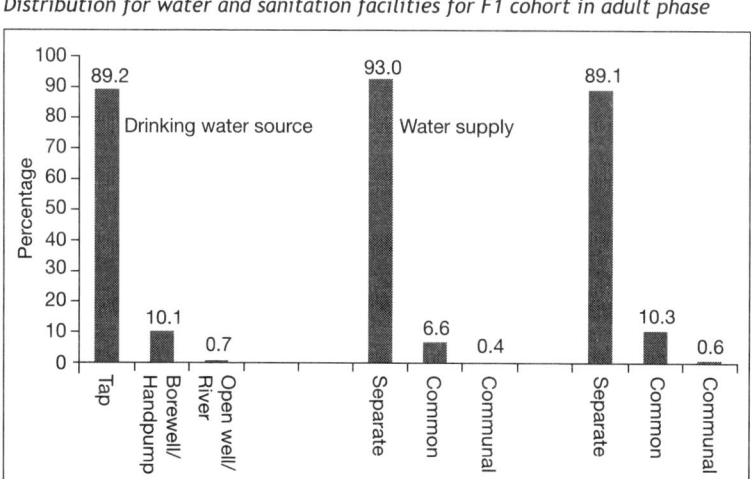

*Source:* Author.

**Figure 4.4.2:**
*Education pattern in F1 cohort in adult phase*

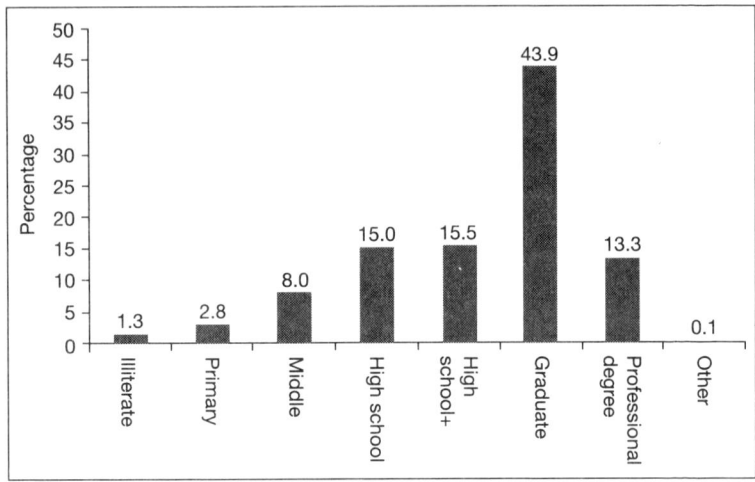

*Source:* Author.

4. **Occupation**

   In the adult phase of 1998–2002, as many as 36.1% were employed in a variety of jobs from teacher to clerk, salesperson, and other professions. The number of unskilled manual labour workers was 1.0%, 14.7% were either skilled manual labour or were self-employed or owned their own business, and 11.8% were class I officers. The housewives were 26.6%. This too was a striking contrast to the childhood phase of 1969–73 when women were mostly homemakers and few were employed in professions. In another change, 18% of the cohorts were doing a secondary business which was mostly of skilled manual labour or small business. Only 4.1% of the cohorts were unemployed (Figure 4.4.3).

5. **Occupation of the Spouses**

   An interesting change was seen in the occupation of spouses. In 39.1%, either of the spouses of the cohort was found working as clerks or teachers. In other professions, 10.5%, were class I officers or a serving officer and 8% were skilled labourers. This pattern was not observed in the earlier phase.

6. **Socio-economic and Wealth Status**

   The wealth or material possession showed 90–99% with electricity fan, radio, television, cable TV, air coolers, electric mixers, and

**Figure 4.4.3:**
*Occupation patterns of F1 cohorts in adult phase*

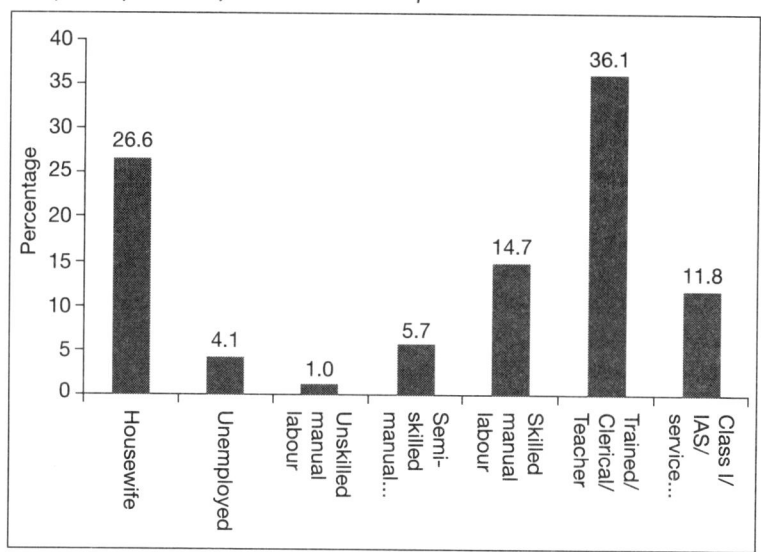

*Source:* Author.

gas stoves. About 80–90% had two wheelers, washing machines, and telephones. About 30–50% had cars and air conditioners and 17.5% had computers at home. This contrasted with earlier phase when the cohort's parents had fans, radios, and scooters and hardly any other possessions.

7. **Social and Cultural Change**

Changes were seen in social life. The women have moved from outdoor household activities such as fetching water and firewood or impounding cattle and go for regular jobs, morning walks in park, yoga in park, exercise, and other leisure activities like watching dramas on television.

A change was also seen in the marriage pattern. Now inter-caste and love marriages were taking place as against exclusive caste-based marriages in the earlier phase.

The cohort and their families spoke 11 languages at home. However, Hindi was the dominant spoken language, with Punjabi in 16%. Many spoke multiple Indian languages.

## Dietary Habits

The dietary habits revealed predominantly non-vegetarian families (60%). Wheat was the most common staple diet as compared to rice.

## Physical Activity

Self-exercise/activity predominated with over 50% walking 1–2.5 km, 20% 3.0–5.0 km, and 22% less than 0.5 km/day. Few used cycling as an exercise. About 58% had mostly sedentary work and 20% were employed with walking or moving around work. Few had a standing profession and hardly any one did hard labour.

## Physical Exercise

Almost 70% did no exercises and 30% did some exercise. The exercise included slow walking in majority (40%) or moderate to brisk walking (33%). Only 10% went for gymnasium and few outdoor games or swimming.

## Smoking and Alcohol

Amongst personal habits, about 80% did not ever smoke. The smoking was seen in 17% and 3% had left smoking. Alcoholic drinks were taken by 32% but a majority of 68% did not take alcohol.

## Medical History

The personal, family, medical, and current and past histories were enquired in over 1,550 cohorts. Surprisingly, a host of illness and/or their history was available in a significant number of cohorts between 26 and 29 years of age and as young adults.

In the current medical illness history, hypertension or high blood pressure was found in 92 or 5.8% of the cases. Tuberculosis was found in 51 or 3.3%, bronchial asthma in 34 or 2.2%, diabetes in 9 or 0.6%, and even stroke was recorded in 2 (0.1%) cases. The other illnesses accounted for less than 10 (1%) with bronchitis and other kind of heart ailments.

Heart-related symptoms were also queried in 1,573 cases and these included breathlessness in 179 (11.4%), chest, jaw/neck, and arm pain in 79 (5%), and discomfort in chest and swollen ankle in 19 (1.2%) each.

Different forms of treatment were being taken for illnesses. For high blood pressure or hypertension, 33 (44.6%) were taking drugs with or without diet control. Salt restriction with diet was being taken by 11 (14.9%). Other treatments included traditional methods with or without diet or salt control and drugs in about 6.7%. Interestingly 1/3rd were taking no treatment.

In eight cases of diabetes, no treatment was being taken in four cases and in other four the patients took traditional, insulin, oral anti-diabetes, or diet control kinds of treatment.

Almost 1/4th or 25.8% of the cohort had by this age suffered from a major illness, injury, or condition causing handicap for life.

The family history for major adult illness was also interesting. Almost 50% had a family history of high blood pressure or hypertension. Almost 1/3rd (36.40%) had a history of diabetes. Angina pectoris or CADs was reported in 1/4 (23.20%) cohorts and stroke by 4%.

The personal history of female cohorts revealed menstrual cycle to be regular in 573 (85%) and irregular in 101 (15%). Only 25 (4%) were using contraceptives and 582 (96%) did not practice any family planning.

One of the interesting studies in the cohorts is related to mental stress and anxiety. This was investigated in over 700 subjects and it revealed findings of concern. Almost 40% of the cohorts felt mental stress, tension, or anxiety. They preferred to keep the stress to themselves in 30% or almost 1/3rd subjects. About 40.7% of the cohort shared it with the families and 11.9% with their friends. Around 5.1% each de-stressed themselves by taking a walk or listening to music.

PART 5

# Childhood Growth, Adult Health, and Human Capital

# 1

# Body Growth, Adult Health, and Disease

## Introduction

The adult phase of the study offered an opportunity to initiate and investigate the influence of maternal health, birth weight, gestation, foetal growth, and body growth through different age periods of childhood and adulthood and their association with adult diseases such as diabetes, metabolic syndrome, and cardiovascular diseases such as hypertension and CAD. It also investigated the relationships of these with human capital development including adult stature, attained schooling, income and wealth generation, and birth weight of the next offspring in the women cohort. The studies were done through new data collection and investigation and/or re-analysis of the data collected in previous studies. The results of this research and analysis have been published in several scientific national and international journals of high impact factor [72]. The parameters which have been used for analysis involved a single factor observation or a collection of several factors expected to influence the outcome.

In almost five decades since its inception, the NDBC has grown and extended to a four generation cohort. At the first contact in 1998, the cohorts had become young adults with their ages varying between 26 and 29 years. By 2015, their ages ranged between 43 and 46 years. During this period, we also investigated the genetic and environmental influences and the trans-generation changes across three generations. We had also shifted our focus to the F2 generation or the children of the cohort for some specific disease patterns.

The description which follows is based on recorded observations which highlight the wealth of the information collected and also provide directions for prevention, early diagnosis, or tracking of chronic adult diseases and possible interventions. Although the studies and publications have extended from the year 1998 to 2017, these are summarised in a cogent, fluent, and consistent manner to maintain continuity and harmony for better understanding and appreciation of the results and inferences and their implications for readers, administrators, policy planners, and health professionals.

(For detailed reading the readers are referred to original publications as listed in the Appendix.)

1. **Size at Birth, Birth Weight, BMI, and Growth in Childhood and Adult Diseases**
   In one of the early publications, we studied about 1,500 subjects who had been followed from preconception to conception, at birth, and then at age-specific periods through childhood to adulthood. Amongst these 23.5% were LBW (birth weight <2,500 g). They were all investigated at 26–29 years of age for prevalence of adult diseases such as diabetes and IGT, hypertension, and others. Half (46%) of them were overweight by international standards and 2/3rd or (66%) by Asian standards. About 10% were obese and central obesity (excessive increase in waist size) was seen in 2/3rd of men and 1/3rd of women.

   The prevalence of IGT was 10.8% and diabetes was 4.2%. Subjects with IGT and diabetes were small in size at birth and up to 2 years of age. They had early rebound of adiposity (this is a natural phenomenon observed as a rise in weight relative to height after 1–2 years of age) and a rapid rise in BMI till adulthood. Interestingly, none of the cohorts were obese between 2 and 12 years of age and only 3.3% of these children were overweight. It was striking that as children these cohorts were thin up to 2 years of age, then gained in weight rapidly, became overweight, and became predisposed to diabetes or glucose balance disturbance at a young adult age. These results also indicated that early rise in BMI or gain in body weight may be a precursor to diabetes or IGT [73].

   The studies demonstrated that by tracking the growth of these children, it is possible to identify individuals who are at risk for developing adult diseases such as diabetes, hypertension, and metabolic syndrome. It showed that the children who have accelerated growth and those who tend to cross upwards in their percentile trajectory are the potential candidates for developing adult diseases such as glucose intolerance, hypertension, metabolic syndrome, and cholesterol aberrations.

Figures 5.1.1–5.1.4 illustrate the observed BMI trajectories from birth till adulthood in various disorders. In all these figures, on Y axis, the BMI Z score of 0 corresponds to the average (or mean) BMI of the cohort subjects at that particular age on the X axis. Figure 5.1.1 shows the BMI trajectory of growth in subjects who developed IGT or diabetes as adults at age of 26–29 years. There was a slight fall in BMI from birth till 3 years of age followed by a persistent rise and the BMI became greater than the population average of the cohort around 10 years of age. Thus, what characterizes the subjects who develop diabetes or IGT is a persistent rise in BMI relative to themselves, and careful growth monitoring can help identify such individuals for intervention.

Similarly, Figure 5.1.2 depicts the longitudinal BMI trajectory in relation to occurrence of higher blood pressure in adulthood. The

**Figure 5.1.1:**
*Longitudinal BMI trajectory in diabetes*

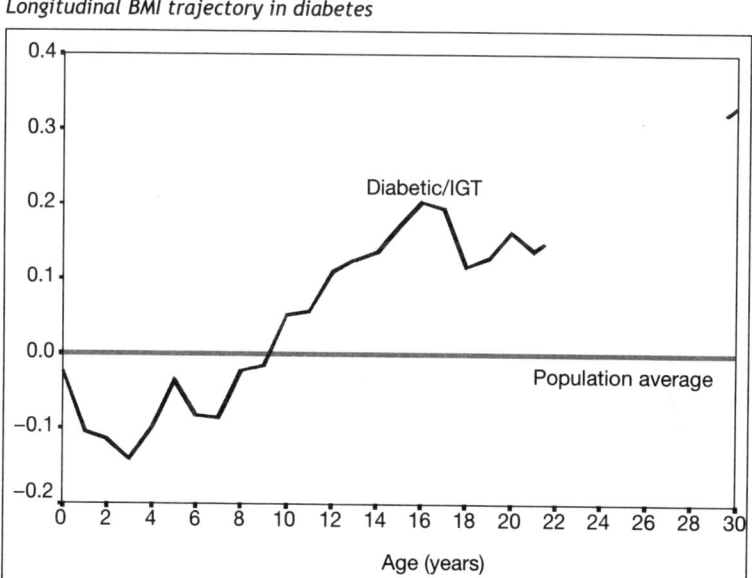

*Source:* NDBC unpublished data.

**Figure 5.1.2:**

*Longitudinal BMI trajectories till adulthood in subjects with high blood pressure, low systolic blood pressure, and low diastolic blood pressure*

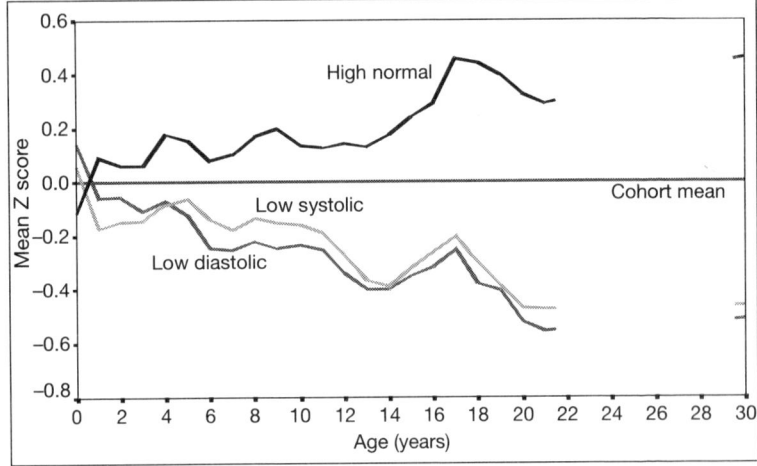

*Source:* NDBC unpublished data.

trends for relative increase in BMI were seen from as early as 2 years of age. It's interesting that predisposition to high blood pressure can be tracked from as early as 2 years of age by longitudinally following BMI Z scores of the population.

The longitudinal BMI trajectories for central obesity (high waist hip ratio) and lipid aberrations (high serum triglycerides) are similarly shown Figures 5.1.3 and 5.1.4. Thus, these studies clearly demonstrated the importance and relevance of growth monitoring during childhood.

2. **Size at Birth, Weight Gain in Infancy and Childhood, and Adult Diabetes Risk**

The NDBC had become part of the COHORT group from four other low- and middle-income countries who had similar cohorts to pool their data and investigate and analyze a spectrum of conditions predisposed by birth weight and body growth in different periods of childhood and its association with adult diseases. In a pooled analysis, the group examined the relationship of birth weight and weight gain in infancy and childhood with predisposition or causation of diabetes and IGT.

**Figure 5.1.3:**
*Longitudinal BMI trajectories till adulthood in subjects with high and low waist hip ratios (high waist hip ratio)*

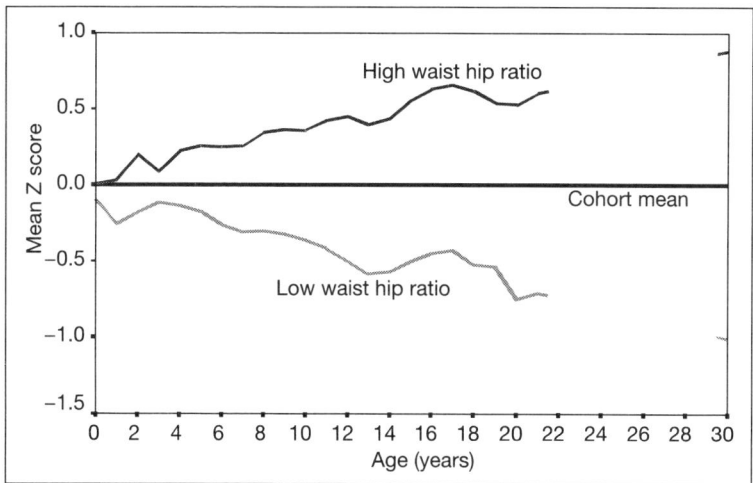

*Source:* NDBC unpublished data.

**Figure 5.1.4:**
*Longitudinal BMI trajectories till adulthood in subjects with high and low serum triglycerides*

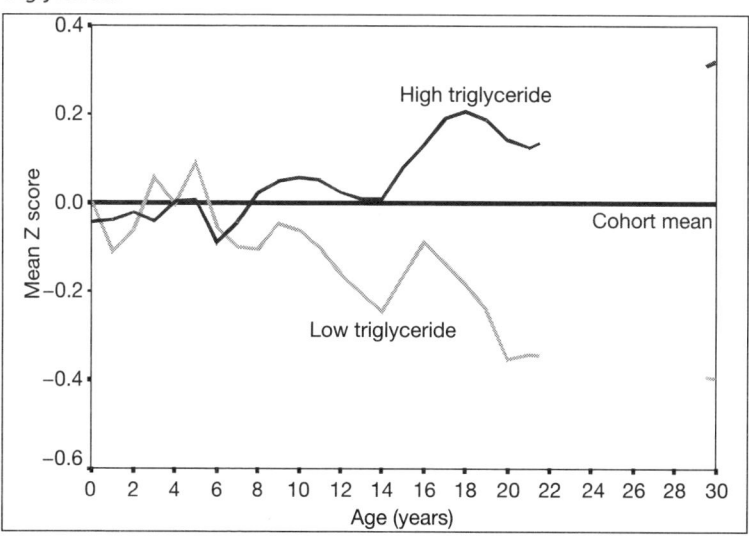

*Source:* NDBC unpublished data.

The growth measurements were analyzed at birth, 12 months, 24 months, 48 months, and young adulthood and their conditional weight gain between these ages and related to adult fasting glucose concentration, risk of glucose intolerance, and insulin resistance. Interesting results were found. It was noted that birth weight had an inverse relationship with adult glucose concentrations and risk of impaired fasting glucose and diabetes mellitus. The greater conditional weight gain (which essentially means higher than expected weight gain between two periods of growth) between 48 months and adulthood was positively associated with glucose concentrations and impaired fasting glucose/diabetes, but no such association was found between birth and at 48 months. This suggested that weight gains or body growth after 4 years need to be closely monitored and its deviations may point to a predisposition to adult diseases. Adult waist circumference was positively associated with early weight gain as well as with adult glucose concentration and impaired fasting glucose/diabetes mellitus. This suggested the relevance and importance of a simple measure like waist circumference, which when associated with early weight gain may suggest onset of glucose metabolism aberrations. Insulin resistance did not record an association with birth weight but greater conditional weight was associated with it [74].

3. **Birth Weight and Type 2 Diabetes**
   The NDBC findings on birth weight were considered for inclusion in a systemic review publication. It showed birth weight to be related to type II diabetes. The association was more in children with LBW (birth weight <2.5 kg). The prevalence of type II diabetes decreased with an increase in birth weight. The literature review further suggested that with an increase in overweight, obesity, and gestational diabetes (diabetes during pregnancy), it is possible that high birth weight may be associated with type II diabetes as is seen some North American native populations. This has been also recently reported from Taiwanese children and adolescence population growing up in a setting where both obesity and type 2 diabetes are common from early age. Maternal diabetes causing an increase in high birth weight may also predispose to diabetes type II occurrence [75].

4. **BMI and Metabolic Syndrome**
   Metabolic syndrome is a disease entity comprising an increase in any of the three factors of abdominal obesity (waist circumference),

triglycerides, high-density lipoprotein (HDL), blood pressure, and fasting glucose. The prevalence of metabolic syndrome was documented to be quite high in the NDBC. The longitudinal BMI trajectories indicated a pattern similar to that observed with other morbidities. However, notably, the relative rise in BMI was evident from birth itself, and also the magnitude of the rise was greater (average rise of 1 Z score as compared to ~0.5 Z score for other morbidities above).

5. **Childhood BMI and Predicting Adult Metabolic Syndrome or Its Components**

It is an established fact that birth weight and child growth have a strong association with the occurrence of IGT and type II diabetes. Any method or test which may help track, predict, or diagnose a risk of diabetes in an individual is, therefore, a public health interest and priority.

The NDBC is a large population-based study. We, therefore, explored the possibility of developing screening methods from childhood body growth measurements to find whether it would help in identifying at risk children for developing adult metabolic syndrome/IGT or diabetes mellitus caused or predisposed by adult adiposity. Our observations suggest that the use of conventional BMI charts are likely to help in identifying children at risk for these diseases if they are followed on BMI charts to detect upward crossing of percentiles and being above the 50th percentile in later measurements. The NDBC proposed BMI charts for tracking adult metabolic syndrome are complex than standard BMI charts and, hence, may be difficult to use in daily practice by clinicians. But the NDBC data strongly brought out the fact that the local population-based reference charts are better and more useful for identifying high risk children than by referring to another population reference chart. Hence, despite being complex, the NDBC charts are likely to be more useful as reference in our population where this needs to be tracked from early childhood [76].

6. **Body Growth and Adult Metabolic Syndrome**

Continuing our interest into the relationship of childhood and adult body growth and body composition, we investigated 1,492 men and women for the occurrence of metabolic syndrome. The prevalence of metabolic syndrome was 29%. It recorded an inverse association with BMI at birth for metabolic syndrome and its components. In infants up to 2 years of age, greater infant

BMI or weight gain was associated with lower risk of diabetes, especially in lower birth weight infants. However, greater infant BMI/weight was associated with an increased risk of metabolic syndrome and its components. The apparent paradox may be due to body composition of different population. In Indian population, a low weight with lean mass is associated with high visceral fat mass or adiposity. In late childhood and adolescence, the NDBC cohort recorded rapid BMI gain and an earlier adiposity rebound which were associated with adult metabolic syndrome and IGT/ diabetes [76].

# 2

# Size at Birth, BMI, Body Composition, and Chronic Adult Diseases

1. **Anthropometric Indicators, Body Composition, and Adult Diseases**
   The Indian population is currently undergoing a transition from undernutrition and underweight to overweight and obesity. As described earlier, this transition predisposes to the development of cardiometabolic diseases. The human body comprises muscle mass (lean mass) or fat mass (adipose tissue). In an overweight or obese person, as defined by the BMI, it is not possible to say whether the increase in BMI is due to excessive increase in muscle or fat mass. We investigated anthropometric or body measurements indicators of body composition in relation to size at birth and serial measurement of BMI in the young NDBC cohort. Almost half the young cohort was overweight and 11% of them were obese by BMI definition.

   The study investigated in both males and females their birth weight, gestational age, foetal growth restriction, BMI, and BMI gain in early childhood, late childhood, adolescence, and adult with body composition broadly used as sum of skin fold thickness from different sites. Interestingly, different patterns were seen for females, and preterm and SGA cohorts (foetal growth restricted). The birth weight was directly related to lean mass. Cohorts with higher birth weight had higher lean mass. In women, only higher birth weight was associated with adiposity (fatness) but not with central obesity (excessively large waist circumference). Higher

BMI and higher BMI gains recorded different patterns. The higher BMI in infancy, childhood, and adolescence was associated with higher adult BMI and higher waist-hip ratio. BMI and BMI gain during infancy and early childhood were more strongly associated with adult lean mass than with adult adiposity or central obesity (large waist circumference). This pattern was more common in males and full term with normal foetal growth.

The contrasting pattern in the first years and later years of childhood and adolescents with rapid gain of BMI and its association with adult diseases strongly suggests the need to monitor and interpret growth patterns during these periods. Our observation suggests that by tracking the BMI pattern and its changes from a lower percentile to a higher percentile is strongly suggestive of a higher risk of overweight and obesity and, hence, for adult disease such as diabetes and hypertension [78].

2. **Birth Weight, Postnatal Weight Gain, and Adult Body Composition**
   The cohort group further evaluated the association between the birth weight, infancy and childhood weight gain, and adult body composition. It used the data for modelling adult body composition as a function of birth weight and conditional weight gain at three age-specific intervals of 0–12 months, 12–24 months, and 24 months-mid childhood.

   The analysis showed that the birth weight was a stronger predictor for fat-free mass than fat mass in adulthood. It was less strong for conditional weight through 24 months and a still lesser or weaker association thereafter. The other inference was that conditional weight at 12 months and mid-childhood were strong predictors of adult body fat percentage. Birth weight in contrast was the weakest predictor.

   The results suggest that birth weight and weight trajectories through 24 months are strongly associated with fat-free mass than fat mass. On the other hand, weight trajectories in mid-childhood predict both fat mass and fat-free mass. Size at birth and weight gain monitoring are, thus, useful tools in assessing body composition [79].

3. **Growth from Birth to Adulthood and Peak Bone Mass and Density**
   We also evaluated the association between longitudinal growth in BMI and bone health in adults. We investigated the size at birth, and changes during 0–2 years, 2–11 years, and 11 years to 20 years in relation to adult BMC and areal and volumetric density in 565

cohorts between the ages of 33 and 39 years. The analysis also considered the adult life factors in relation to bone measurement, size and growth in early life. Measurements were obtained for femoral neck, lumbar spine, and forearm bone. The BMC, areal bone mineral density (aBMD), and spine and femoral neck (vBMD) were measured using dual X-ray absorptiometry (DEXA). Birth length and height and weight gain during infancy, childhood, and adolescence were positively correlated with adult BMC at all sites except for birth length and femoral neck.

The results further showed independent influence of birth weight and postnatal growth in bone mass in young adults of either sex. Bone size was strongly related to height and weight at birth and height growth during infancy. The measure of bone density was strongly related to BMI and BMI gain during childhood and adolescence [80].

4. **Body Growth and Maresh Reference Data**

Stunting is a major public health problem in India and other developing countries of South East Asia. The availability of prospective age-specific data on body growth in supine position to standing height prompted us to compare the Maresh reference data with WHO international standards for normal growth in healthy children. We undertook the analysis as there were no published studies comparing the Maresh reference data with a growth standard. The WHO multicentre growth reference study (MGRS) group published the growth standard of children who apparently grew in optimal conditions. The publication discusses the merits of the Maresh data vis-á-vis WHO growth standard and highlights that Maresh reference data may not be as useful for identifying stunting and for estimating stunting prevalence in prehistoric populations. It further points to the possibility of statural growth being a reflection of health environmental difference rather than ethnic or population difference. It also suggested the Maresh reference data to be more suitable for estimating age and body size in healthy children from femoral length [81].

5. **Cardiovascular Diseases**

a. **Childhood BMI and adult pro-inflammatory and pro-thrombotic risk factors**

Our country is expected to have increasing morbidity and mortality due to cardiovascular diseases in the future. LBW and excessive weight gain or obesity is known to predispose to cardiovascular disease. The NDBC had a high prevalence (26.2%) of LBW rate. We evaluated one of the hypothesized mechanisms of increased cardiometabolic morbidity and mortality, namely, pro-inflammatory and pro-thrombotic risk factors in adulthood in relation to longitudinal BMI growth.

The association of birth weight, BMI at 2 years and through childhood to adulthood was related to adult pro-inflammatory and pro-thrombotic risk factors including high-sensitivity C-reactive protein (hsCRP), fibrinogen, and with plasminogen activator inhibitor-I (PAI-1) in 1,583 subjects. It was noted that an inverse relationship existed between birth weight and BMI at birth and 2 years for hsCRP in both sexes; with fibrinogen in women and BMI at 2 years with PAI-1 concentration in men. Greater BMI gain between 2 and 11 years of age and/or 11 years and adulthood was associated with increase in all pro-inflammatory and pro-thrombotic markers. These associations diminished after adjusting for adiposity. The study suggested that birth weight and BMI gain between 2 and 11 years of age and adulthood had an association with cardiovascular risk markers [82].

b. **Body growth and body composition, cardiovascular risk factors, and incidence of cardiometabolic risk factors**
One of the major objectives of adult studies was to find the incidence (rate of development) of cardiovascular diseases and risk factors affecting them. The first phase of the study was between the years 1998 and 2002 and the next phase from 2006 to 2009. The age of the cohort was respectively 29 ±1 years in the first phase and 36 ±1 years in the second phase. The risk factors which were assessed included BMI, waist circumference, hip circumference, systolic blood pressure, diastolic blood pressure, blood cholesterol, HDL and low-density lipoprotein (LDL) cholesterol levels, and triglycerides.

The annual incidence for obesity was 2.0% in men and 2.2% for women. The hypertension annual incidence in men was 4.2% and in female it was 1.8%. The diabetes annual incidence in men was 1.0 and in women 0.5%. The IGT and diabetes prevalence significantly increased in the interval of 6–8 years in two phases. The IGT increased from 10% to 14% and the diabetes doubled from 5% to 12% in men and from 3.5% to 7% in women. A significant association was also found between these two periods for increase in waist circumference, waist hip ratio, total cholesterol, and triglycerides. The total cholesterol increased in both men and women. The LDL cholesterol did not change in either sex but the HDL cholesterol increased in both sexes and was slightly at higher level for woman.

In general, women showed higher rate of increase in obesity but men predominated in hypertension and diabetes while central obesity was noted in both. The alarming increase in the rate of the cardiovascular risk factors, diabetes, and hypertension could be due to the NDBC going through a transitional period of nutrition, greater affluence, and improvement in environment. Other significant contributory factors could be the change in lifestyle, the increases in wealth and assets, sedentary habits and diet [83].

c. **Body growth and body composition and predictors of carotid intima-media thickness and carotid plaques**
In 2006–09, we focused on investigating carotid intima media thickness (CIMT; thickness of wall of the blood vessels supplying brain) and carotid plaques which are the precursors of atherosclerosis. We related these to anthropometry, metabolic syndrome, lipid profile, blood pressure, and others. Around 600 NDBC cohorts with mean age of 36 years participated in the study. B mode carotid ultrasound was done. Carotid plaques were present in 33% of men and 36% of women. A positive association with waist circumference was found with both. Longer body length at 2 year was significantly associated with CIMT. A higher diastolic blood pressure, triglycerides, PAI-I, insulin resistance, metabolic syndrome, and lower HDL were associated with CIMT. The data suggested that it is possible to identify at risk adult for abnormal CIMT by observing early growth, socio-economic status, and CVS risk factors [84].

6. **Infant Feeding and Adult Health and Outcome**

a. **Infant feeding and cardiovascular risk factors young adults**
Exclusive and prolonged breastfeeding has been known to have protective benefits for child in prevention of diseases in early life and development of chronic adult disease. There are enough studies to show the benefits in reduction of immediate and long-term morbidities. The COHORT group investigated the benefits of breastfeeding and no breastfeeding,

late introductions of complementary feeding and influence on three major adult diseases of blood pressure, obesity and diabetes. It showed no difference in systolic blood pressure in the groups which were initially breastfed and in those who were not initially breastfed. The duration of breastfeeding recorded an inverse relationship with overweight or obesity. The cohorts who were breastfed for longer duration had thinner skin folds but this was significant only after confounder adjustments. The most interesting finding was timing of introduction of complementary food. It showed that later introduction of complementary food reduced adult adiposity. However, this study failed to demonstrate a definite positive benefit of breastfeeding on three major adult diseases of hypertension, diabetes, and/or over weight and obesity [85].

b. **Infant feeding practices and school attainment**

The positive influences of breastfeeding for immediate and long-term benefits are well known. Amongst, the several advantages, improved cognitive performance has been reported mostly from the well-developed countries, which investigated exclusive breastfeeding for first 6 months vis-á-vis intellectual development. The COHORTS group from the low and middle-income countries explored the association between exclusive breastfeeding and the time of introduction of complementary feeding with achieved schooling. A total of 10,082 young adults of the five cohorts participated in the study. The exposures studied included ever breastfed, duration of breastfeeding, and introduction of complementary food to successfully completing the highest grade of schooling.

The analysis of breastfeeding association recorded heterogeneous data. It did not record a clear positive association with schooling. Similarly, the ever-breastfeeding group also recorded inconsistent observations across all five cohorts. The duration of breastfeeding too had similar observations.

Our findings of lack of association between breastfeeding and schooling are in contrast to other reports, which record consistent performance with intelligence test in breastfed infants. This data suggest the possibility that the early advantage accrued in intelligence performance is of shorter than expected period and does not last long in later life. It also does not result in higher schooling achievement. It is possible that many more factors other than breastfeeding may be responsible for schooling [86].

# 3

# Body Growth and Human Capital Development

1. **Growth Pattern in Early Childhood and Attained Stature**
   Stunting in childhood and adult life are considered indicators of human capital development. In an earlier publication, we had shown that stunting at 2 years is related to attainment of final stature and income generation. In further analysis, the cohort group analyzed the influence of length at birth at age 12 months, 24 months, and mid-childhood by constructing individual cohort and sex-specific conditional length measures in 4,659 individuals' pooled analysis. The analysis revealed that individuals for all cohorts site experienced growth failure of varying degree, with the maximal disadvantage in height for age Z score at 24 months. Adult height showed a strong association with length at birth and conditional length at 24 months of age. Adult stature was influenced by growth failure in first year [87].

2. **Weight Gain in the First Two Years of Life is an Important Predictor of Schooling Outcome**
   The association between birth weight and weight gain in first 2 years (0–24 months) and 2–4 years (24–48 months) with schooling outcome including age at entry, any time grade failure, and completing schooling was also investigated by the cohorts group. Birth weight, weight gain in 0–24 months and 24–48 months, and the occurrence of stunting at 2 years significantly influenced the schooling outcome such as enrolment age in the school, failure in any grades or class during schooling, and completing the school

education. One SD increase in weight gain between birth and 24 months increased the schooling by 0.9 years. This, in turn, is expected to directly influence the likely increase in the income over a life time period by about 10%. An increase in birth weight showed an increase in schooling years and decreased the chances of a failure in any grade or class at any time during schooling by about 8%. Thus, a weight gain in the first 2 years and a higher birth weight influenced school education by decreasing the chances of a failure in any grade or completing school education. This results in decreasing chances of a decline in income. Weight gain in children born small (LBW or SGA) is likely to improve schooling even better than normal weight infants [88].

3. **Association of Linear Growth and Relative Weight Gain During Early Life with Adult Health and Human Capital**

The influence of birth weight, weight gain, and linear growth at different periods of childhood on survival and development of adult diseases such as metabolic syndrome, diabetes, and cardiovascular disorders was investigated in the five cohorts by the group.

In a pooled analysis, 8,362 individuals participated who had at least one outcome measure. The different outcome measures varied from cohort's gestation to birth size to adult anthropometry, body composition, blood pressure, schooling, maternal height, glucose haemostasis, stunting, and others. Several features were noted. These showed that a higher birth weight was associated with a higher BMI and decreased risk of short adult stature. It also had decreased chances of not completing secondary school education. Similarly, faster gain in height strongly decreased the risk of short adult stature and the chances of not completing secondary education. However, it increased the risks of overweight and blood pressure. The results further showed that a faster relative body weight gain was associated with risk of overweight and elevated blood pressure. It also suggested that linear growth and relative weight gain are not associated with glucose disturbance and that higher birth weight decreased the risk of dysglycemic disorder [89].

4. **Preterm, Small for Gestation, and Adult Human Capital and Outcome**

One of the main interests of the NDBC research has been to find the outcome and sequelae of LBW which comprise preterm and growth restricted or SGA infants. In the cohort study, we investigated 4,517 adults for the association of postnatal growth patterns with adult height, blood pressure, glucose, and schooling attainment. The SGA in this group were almost twice the number of preterms.

SGA were shorter in stature than preterm when both were compared to term normal AGA adults. The SGA measured 2.43 cm less and the preterm 1.19 cm less as compared to term AGA. The blood pressure and glucose did not differ in the two groups, but the schooling attainment was 0.46 year lower in preterm and 0.42 year lower in those born term but SGA as compared to those born term-AGA. In brief, being born early or with growth restriction may be detrimental to final attainment of stature and scholastic performance [90].

5. **Parental Childhood Growth and Offspring Birth Weight**
Parental body growth and stature may influence the offspring growth and height. The influence of parental growth at birth and age specific periods through adulthood was investigated to find the relationship with offspring birth weight. The study in a sense aimed at parental anthropometry to predict birth weight of the offspring.

Paternal birth weight and linear growth from birth to 2 years was associated with birth weight but the later growth beyond the 2 year period was not related to offspring birth weight. In contrast, maternal growth in first 2 years was not associated with birth weight but was significantly related from 2 years to mid-childhood and mid-childhood to adulthood. The study points to the relevance of nutrition in first 2 years for the father or male gender and nutritional care of the mother from 2 years and beyond. It is known that pre-pregnancy nutritional state of the mother affects the foetal growth and birth weight [91].

# 4

# Parental Influences on Adult Health

1. **Maternal Height and Child Growth Patterns from Intrauterine Period to Adulthood**
   The influence of maternal health and well-being on her off spring is well documented and the effect could manifest anytime from preconception to conception and/or during the childhood period. The COHORT group investigated specifically the influence of the maternal height on the offspring intrauterine growth, growth from birth to 2 years, 2 years to mid-childhood, and mid-childhood to adulthood. Pooled analysis was done in 7,605 mothers in whom this data/information was available. Maternal height influenced the child from foetal period through birth and childhood to adulthood. The influence is more marked in later childhood than in early childhood. Offspring were taller than their mothers. Maternal height was associated with birth weight, birth height, and conditional height examined at each age. The data also suggested that while maternal height influences the offspring's linear growth, it is being driven both by genetic and non-genetic factors such as nutrition, environment, and socio-economic status [92].

2. **Maternal and Child Undernutrition**
   Maternal and child undernutrition are a common occurrence in several parts of the world, especially South East Asia, America, and Africa. The COHORT group investigated the influence of maternal size, birth weight, foetal growth restriction, and the individual's weight, height, and BMI at 2 years of age and related these to selected adult outcomes which included final attained

height, schooling, income generation, and birth weight of the next offspring.

Growth failure, which occurred in the intrauterine period and in the first two years significantly influenced the attainment of final height but was mostly inconsequential thereafter. Growth failure in the period 12–24 months is less predictive of adult stature than growth failure occurring at birth or in the first year of life. These observation are perhaps more specific than similar earlier reports of growth failure occurring at different periods of childhood in influencing the final attainment of adult height.

An analysis was also done for determining the influence of birth weight and weight gain during 0–24 and 24–48 months for higher grade attainment, grade failure, and age at school entry. The results showed that weight gain during 0–24 months had the strongest influence on schooling outcomes. These were followed by birth weight. Weight gain during 24–48 months had the least influence on schooling outcome. A most interesting and significant finding was the association of maternal undernutrition with lower birth weight on next generation offspring.

The observations that growth failure in the intrauterine period, the first 12 months, and to a lesser extend in 12–24 months influences the major component of human capital development of adult height, schooling, earning capacity, and birth weight of next offspring perhaps led to the coining of the currently popular term of the 'first 1,000 days'.

The results of this analysis are of considerable interest, relevance, and importance for caregivers, administrators, and professionals involved in maternal and child health, nutrition, and policy planning. The findings have a direct message for policy formulation of maternal and child nutrition [93].

3. **Association Between Maternal Age at Childhood and Child and Adult Outcome in the Offspring**

Teenage and late age pregnancies are known to influence the foetal and newborn outcome. In a COHORTS group study, we determined the impact of young age (<19 years) and advanced maternal age (>35 years) on selective offspring outcomes, encompassing childhood and adulthood. These included birth weight, gestational age, height for age, weight for height Z score in childhood, and attained schooling, adult height, body composition, and cardiometabolic risk factors as adults. About 22,188 mothers were analyzed; the criterion being at least one of the outcomes being available for analysis.

Young mothers of less than 19 years were prone to have LBW, preterm births, stunting at 2 years, short adult height, poor schooling, and higher adult fasting glucose concentration. These disadvantages were unaffected by socio-economic status, height, breastfeeding, duration, and parity. Older mothers above 35 years age had children who were at risk of preterm births and glucose disturbance. The other disadvantages as mentioned for younger mother were greatly reduced. Elder mothers had children with greater height and better schooling. Maternal age, except for glucose, was unrelated to other cardiometabolic risk factors [94].

# 5

# Body Growth, Genetic Studies, and Adult Health Outcome

The NDBC is currently a four-generation study. It had over the last four decades gathered considerable information influencing socio-cultural aspects, economic and educational status, environmental changes, nutritional patterns, and lifestyle changes in the cohort, its families, and population. We had tried to study the impact of these changes on the body growth, body composition, and their association with chronic diseases. It was, therefore, natural for us to also investigate the influence and links if any with genetic markers of the body.

1. **Serial Changes in Childhood Body Mass Index and Coronary Artery Disease Risk Factor and their Relationship of APOA5, PPAR gamma, and HL Gene Variants**

   Triglycerides are an independent risk factor for CAD, and this is especially important in Indians because of high prevalence of hypertriglyceridemia. Both genetic and environmental factors determine triglyceride levels. In our earlier NDBC studies, we had recorded hypertriglyceridemia in 41% of men and 11% of women. Subjects who had high triglycerides had more rapid BMI or weight gain than rest of the cohort throughout infancy, childhood, and adolescence. We analyzed polymorphisms in re-sequencing the apolipoprotein A5 (APOA5), hepatic lipase, and peroxisome proliferator-activated receptor gamma (*PPARγ*) genes and investigated their association with birth weight and serial changes in BMI. We assessed whether these polymorphisms influenced lipid and other variables and serial changes in BMI, both individually and together.

The results of this study had suggested that birth weight and serial changes in anthropometry from birth to adulthood do not have any significant relationship with the polymorphism in *APOA5*, PPARγ, and hepatic lipase. The promoter polymorphism in *APOA5* is associated with a raised serum triglyceride levels; the age, gender, and BMI-adjusted effect size being substantial (23 mg/dl). The promoter polymorphism in hepatic lipase is associated with higher HDL2 levels. An interaction between polymorphisms in *APOA5* and hepatic lipase seems to influence the serum triglyceride levels which need to be further explored [95].

2. **Phenotypic Characterization of Diabetes in a Young Delhi Cohort: Association with Low Birth Weight**

This project had aimed to investigate the autoimmune disease markers of diabetes, such as generalized anxiety disorder (GAD) and islet antigen 2 (IA-2) in the NDBC subjects to understand the phenotypic character of diabetes in the cohort. An attempt was also made for correlation of the levels of these markers with the birth weight, ponderal index, BMI, and BMI trajectories and finally correlation of these markers with glucose, insulin, insulin resistance, and B-cell function. The phenotypic character of IGT and diabetes mellitus was characterized in relation to autoimmune disease markers, namely, insulin antibodies GAD and IA-2. Insulin antibodies had no relationship to childhood body size (birth weight, ponderal index, and BMI) or growth (BMI) trajectories. There was evidence of insulopenic association with both antibodies (IA and GAD). This was considered as a biological expectation.

3. **Genetic Determinants of Birth Weight and Growth Trajectory and Influence of Parental Genotype on these Anthropometric Indicators**

Birth-weight and early life growth patterns are believed to be major predictors of inflammatory state, type 2 diabetes, and cardiovascular disease. We are trying to investigate whether birth weight and growth trajectory, which predicts progressive changes in inflammatory state, are genetically determined. It is hoped that recognition of such genetic factors may help in understanding mechanisms involved in early growth and development and could lead to formulation of newer strategies to prevent adult metabolic disorders. This study is in progress and is expected to be completed in near future.

4. **Relationship of Birth Size and Infant and Childhood Growth to Telomere Length in Adulthood**

A telomere is the end of a chromosome. Telomeres are made of repetitive sequences of non-coding DNA that protect the chromosome from damage. Each time a cell divides, the telomeres become shorter. It protects the end of the chromosome from deterioration or from fusion with neighbouring chromosomes. The telomeres are disposable buffers at the ends of chromosomes, which are truncated during cell division; their presence protects the genes before them on the chromosome from being truncated instead. Over time, due to each cell division, the telomere ends become shorter. They are replenished by an enzyme, telomerase reverse transcriptase.

Dynamic biochemical environment, early life exposures, metabolic health, chronic stress, and socio-demographic factors can all potentially regulate an individual's telomere length from conception to death. Early life exposure due to women's nutritional status during pregnancy, which is reflected in the birth weight of the infant and the subsequent catch up growth during early childhood, has been linked to obesity and metabolic diseases later in life. Animal studies have provided some evidence on the effect of foetal programming on telomere length. Our interest in this study arose due to very few studies, which have compared telomere length in LBW children against normal birth weight children. The NDBC, with birth weight and subsequent growth being tracked, provided an excellent opportunity to corroborate the findings in humans and is likely to provide a mechanistic link between early growth and adult metabolic diseases.

We, therefore, proposed the study of telomere length in young adults of the NDBC and their relation to birth weight and serial changes in BMI (at different stages of growth). We also propose to correlate the telomere length with other cardiovascular risk factors. The study is still in progress.

# PART 6

# Intergenerational and Trans-generational Studies

# Introduction

## *The Four Generations of New Delhi Birth Cohort*

The NDBC is currently in its 5th decade and 47th year of follow-up. It has blossomed into a four-generation family cohort. The F0 are the parents of the cohort; F1 are the NDBC themselves; F2 generation are the children of the NDBC; and F3 are the grandchildren of the NDBC.

The last census of the NDBC family was started in September 2015 and is still ongoing. In the F1 generation or the NDBC, we have 2,105 cohorts currently available with males being 1,103 and females being 1,002. The F0 generation includes parents of the F1 cohort and currently has 1,775 subjects. Amongst these, 941 F1 cohort subjects have both parents alive, 660 cohorts have only their mothers alive, and 174 are single fathers of the cohorts who are alive.

In the F2 generation, we have 3,572 children. Amongst these, 1,938 are boys and 1,634 are girls. In the male F2 children, 992 are sons born to male cohorts and 930 are sons born to female cohorts. In the F2 female children, 835 are daughters of male cohorts and 799 are daughters of female cohorts. The fourth generation number only 9, with 5 males and 4 females (Figure. 6.0.1).

It is interesting to note that in the F0 generation more fathers had died as compared to mothers. This suggested early deaths in males, while females had a longer life. In the F1 generation of the NDBC, the sex ratio of the cohorts was almost the same. But in the F2 generation, there is slight preponderance of males (54%). Even in the children of the F2 of either sex, males seem to be larger in numbers. There seemed to be an apparent change in sex preference by the F1 generation cohort parents in favour of a male child as compared to a female child. This trend is consistent with that seen in national and Delhi state's recent census.

**Figure 6.0.1:**
*The four generations of the NDBC*

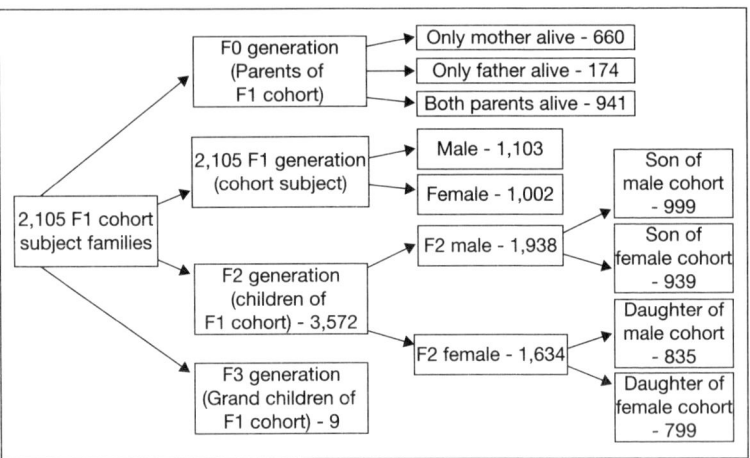

*Source:* Author.

# 1

# The Intergenerational Change in F1 and F2 Generation

1. **Anthropometry**

   The NDBC and their family members who accompanied them to the field clinics were measured as per the protocol for F1. While no special or age specific efforts were made to invite F0 and F2 generations to attend clinics with F1, they were always welcomed and encouraged to attend. Sometimes there were concurrent projects on F0 and F2 generations, and hence extra efforts were made to persuade them to attend the clinics. The F0 mostly did not come to the clinic and their measurements were obtained at home.

   The anthropometric measurements were obtained in about 1,500 F2 children of F1 subjects. Growth charts were generated for weight, height, and BMI for F1 generation using longitudinal measurements and LMS Cole's approach. These charts were used to compute age- and gender-specific Z score for F2 generation. The F1 generation Z score was interpolated using neighbouring measurements at the exact age of the F2 measurement. The window used for F1 interpolation was within 0.5 years (up to 1 year), 1 year (1–2 years), 1.5 years (2–3 years), and 2 years (all ages after 3 years). The intergenerational change (F2–F1) was compared among five age groups including 0–5, 5–7.5, 7.5–10, 10–12.5, and > 12.5 years of age.

   The positive intergenerational change in anthropometric Z score according to age is shown in Figure 6.1.1. A positive change

**Figure 6.1.1:**
*Intergenerational changes in anthropometry*

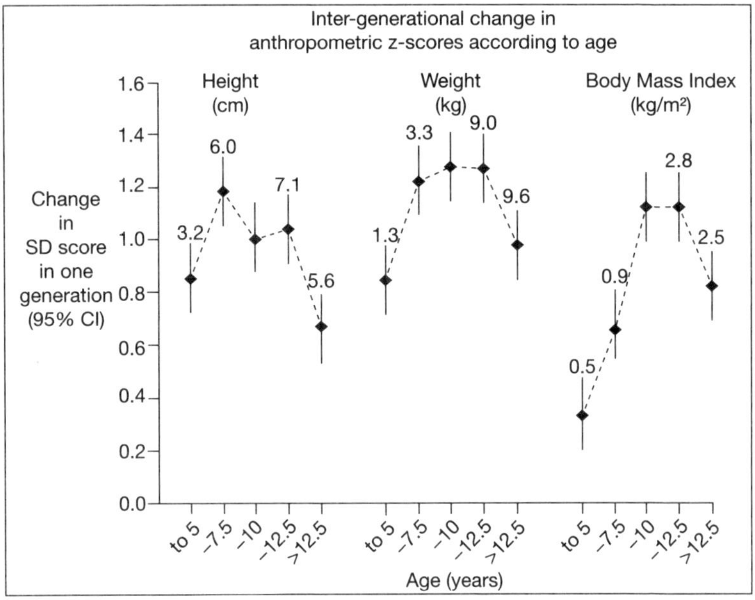

Source: NDBC data, unpublished.

was observed in SD scores at all ages for height, weight, and BMI. The change in height measured from 0.7–1.2 SD (2.7 to 8.1 cm). The change in weight was from 0.8 to 1.3 SD (1.0 to 10.7 kg), and the change for BMI was from 0.3 to 1.1 SD (0.5 to 2.9 kg/m²). The maximum change for BMI was observed between 7.5 and 12.5 years and for the height it was seen between 5 and 12.5 years of age. There was a positive association of the intergenerational change with the current (at the time of F2 measurement) parental education and wealth (Figure 6.1.1).

The results of the intergenerational change are very interesting. It shows a gain in all the measurements suggesting a positive generational change. This change has happened in the same family, living in the same but improved environment, nutrition, and income. No active intervention was done and this change can be regarded as a natural happening over a period of one generation. The positive association with parental education and wealth suggests that these may have also influenced the intergeneration change.

2. **Intergenerational Change on Birth Weight and Low Birth Weight Prevalence**

Birth weight and LBW have been the focus of various studies and analysis of the NDBC project. We had observations for both F1 generation of the NDBC and their children (F2 generation) on birth weight and the prevalence of LBW. Hence, it was considered prudent to compare the change in the two generations which came from the same surroundings, environment, and culture, but almost after three decades of each other.

The mean birth weight was shown to be marginally higher by 32.8 g in the parents of the NDBC (F1 generation) as compared to their children or F2 generation (F1 = 2850.06 ± 417.71 g; F2 = 2817.22 ± 517.78 g). This was a surprising finding as the general environment, hygiene, nutrition, education, sanitation, maternal health, and pregnancy care were distinctly better for the F2 generation than their parents or F1 generation. But the changes in the overall situation particularly for maternal health and other socio-environmental change for the next F2 generation was seen in the prevalence of the LBW children. This declined from 20.8% in the F1 generation to 18.0% in the F2 generation. In general, otherwise the weight distribution pattern in different birth weight groups of 500 g each remained the same. The findings are not surprising as birth weight is influenced by a host of factors from socio-economic, environment to mother's health, nutritional status prior to pregnancy, and during pregnancy, pregnancy care, and complications (Figure. 6.1.2).

This is again a significant finding as in the NDBC population no specific maternal, health, or other intervention was done for improving the birth weight for F2 children. The change thus may be due to social, economic, and environmental improvement between the two generations.

3. **Malnutrition**

**Intergeneration changes in the malnutrition status of the New Delhi Birth Cohort**

Nutrition has always been of prime concern in the NDBC studies. We have recorded a significant intergenerational change in the socio-cultural, economic, education, and environment in the NDBC. While we did not record the dietary and physical activity change in detail, a transition was visible in nutritional habits due to abundance of different kinds of food and their ready availability

**Figure 6.1.2:**
*Birth weight and LBW intergenerational change*

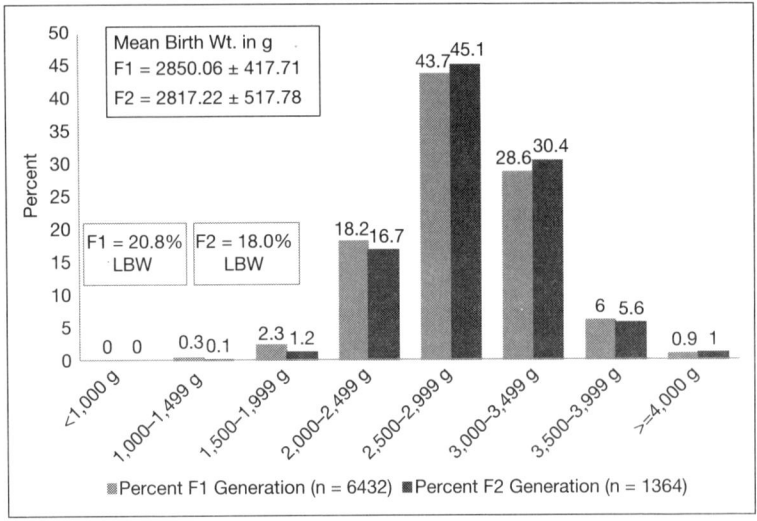

*Source:* Author.

We have been collecting data in the two generations the F1 generation of the NDBC and F2 generation-the children of the NDBC cohort for nutritional assessment. A comparison was done in the two generations. Undernutrition was assessed from birth to five years and overnutrition or overweight and BMI from early childhood period to adolescence.

a. **Wasting**

The prevalence of wasting decreased in F2 in the first 3 years, being striking in the first and second years, but increased in the fourth and fifth years (Figure 6.1.3). The decline in the first year happened from 10.4% to 3.3% and in the second year from 9.2% to 5.3%. In the third year, the decline was very small, but in the fourth and fifth years, wasting increased by about 1%. This was unexpected and needs to be confirmed and investigated (Figure 6.1.3).

b. **Stunting**

Stunting in F2 decreased throughout the first five years as compared to the F1 generation. This was sharp in the first two years where it decreased 50–66%, and thereafter it was 30–50% (Figure 6.1.4).

**Figure 6.1.3:**
*Prevalence of wasting in F1 and F2 generation*

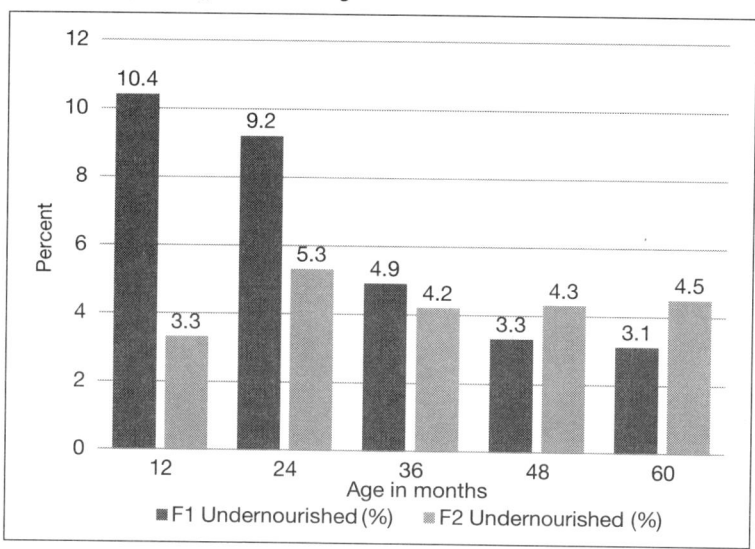

*Source:* Author.

**Figure 6.1.4:**
*Prevalence of stunting in F1 and F2 generations*

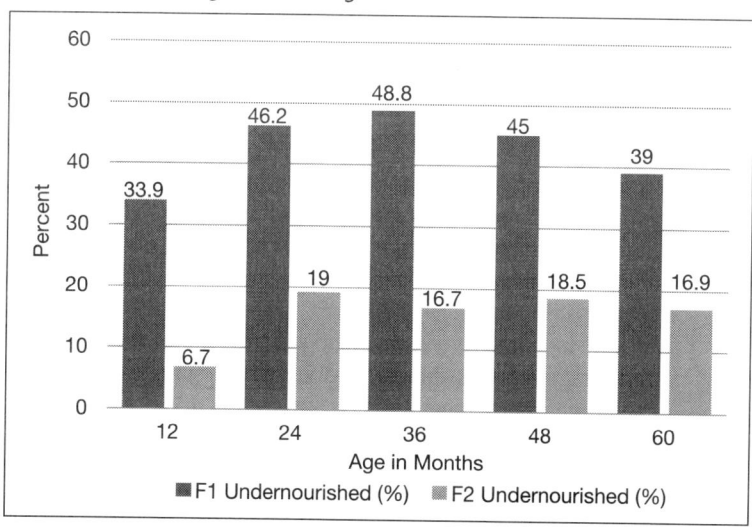

*Source:* Author.

**Figure 6.1.5:**
*Prevalence of underweight in F1 and F2 generations*

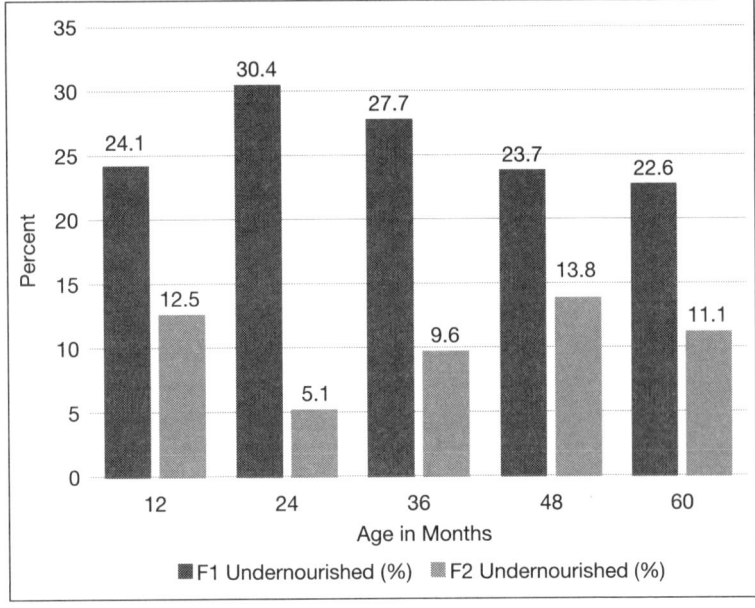

*Source:* Author.

This is a very heartening finding as India is struggling with the problem of stunting, which has consequences for later life. The improved condition could be due to better environment, maternal health, and nutrition but may also be an intergenerational change.

c. **Underweight**

The prevalence of underweight also showed a uniform decline in the F2 generation as compared to the F1 generation. The decline was sharp in the second year and decreased by almost six times in the second year. In the remaining years, the decline happened in the range of 30–50%. (Figure 6.1.5). The general decline in all the five years could be due to improved nutrition and less infections due to health practices and environment sanitation improvement. The sharp decline in the second year is difficult to explain (Figure 6.1.5).

d. **Body Mass Index**

The BMI in F1 and F2 generations have been compared in the scatter plot. This shows an early rise from early childhood and remains scattered throughout (Figure 6.1.6). This is of concern as overweight and obesity are emerging as a public health problem from early childhood to adolescence.

The changes in the undernutrition status, especially stunting are heartening. These are perhaps reflective of the overall change which has come in the NDBC population. These changes include social, cultural, environmental, educational, and wealth status. The national programme and increasing awareness, childhood immunization, and decrease in infection rates and availability of better medical facilities may have collectively helped decrease undernutrition prevalence and stunting.

Overweight in F2 generation was observed from infancy and continued to be seen throughout the childhood and adolescence. It also appeared to increase with an increase in age. This was strikingly different as compared to F1 generation in whom overweight was seen from the age of 5 years and was uniformly observed at different ages from childhood to adolescence. The emergence of overweight and obesity is directly related to lifestyle changes including affluence, lack of physical activity, TV viewing, computer time, and nutrition with availability of fast food and others. The continued undernutrition and overnutrition are the double burden of nutrition, which the country is now facing.

4. **Trans-generation Sleep Disorders in the Three Generations of NDBC**

The adult phase of the NDBC has been largely focused on the cardiometabolic and related adult diseases and their relationship with body growth and body composition. In recent years, sleep disorders and disturbances have been linked or found associated with cardiovascular stroke and diabetes. The NDBC is now an extensive depository of data on factors contributing to these disorders. A study was therefore planned to investigate the sleep and its association with cardiometabolic risk factors in the three generations of the NDBC cohort. It is well known that sleep patterns may be influenced by the family culture, habits, and lifestyles.

The study involved the three generations of the NDBC. The F0 generation are the parents of the cohort, F1 generation are the NDBC cohorts, and F2 generation are the children of the NDBC cohort. F2 generation or the children were further divided into two groups of 4–12 years and 12–18 years as these are known to behave differently. In each group, there were more than 200 subjects.

**Figure 6.1.6:**
*Scatter graph of BMI change in F1 and F2 generations*

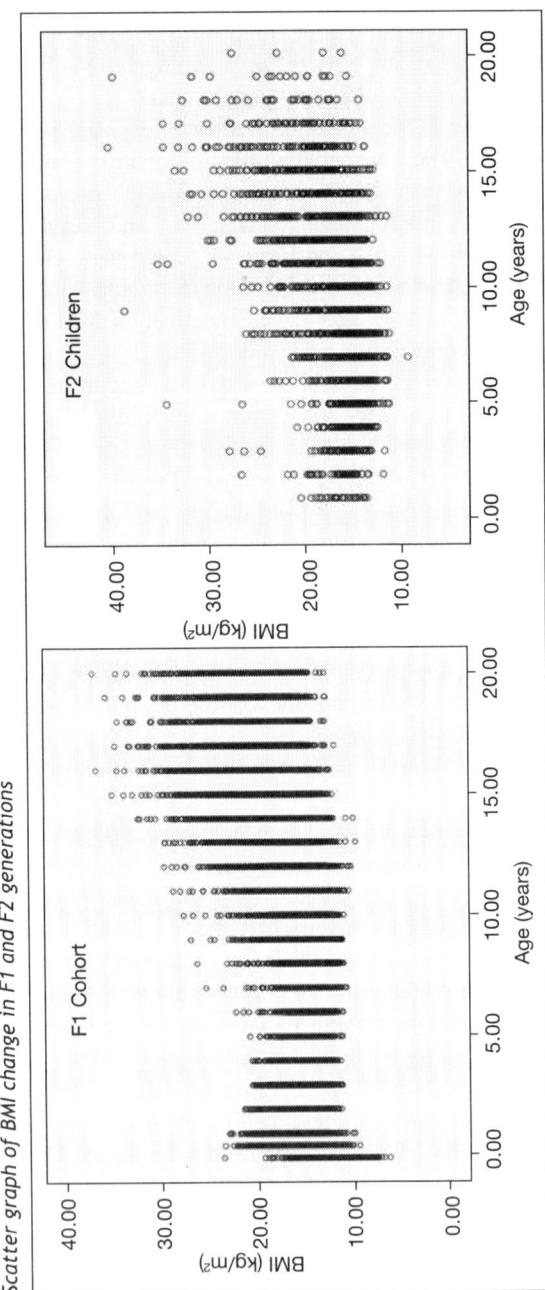

*Source:* Author.

Amongst the three generations, the grandparents slept the least number of hours and even in them the grandmothers slept the least. The F2 generation slept the maximum. The sleep duration seemed to decrease with an increase in age. The grandparents slept for about 6–7 hours and the children slept the most with about 9 hours of sleep.

All adult diseases seemed to increase with age. Hypertension, obesity, and dyslipidaemia were the most frequent adult health disorders. Obesity in older generations of F0 was seen in 36.6% of grandmothers, 17.1% of grandfathers, and 22.4% of the F1 NDBC cohorts. In the F0 generation, in both grandparents, hypertension was seen in 60%; in F1 generation it was observed in 25%; and in the youngest generation or the children F2 generation it was noted in 12.1% (Tables 6.1.1 and 6.1.2).

High cholesterol levels were more frequent in the fathers of F1 generation as compared to other members in other generations. It was seen in all three generations but was more common in F0 and F1 as compared to F2 generation. A similar pattern was also observed for triglyceride levels in all the generations.

Amongst the sleep disorders, the F0 and F1 generations most commonly suffered from hypersomnia, followed by insomnia and then parasomnia. Grandmothers had the highest number of sleep problem. The F0 and F1 had problems in sleep initiation but it was more common in the F0 grandparent generation.

The females in all three generations slept the least. Snoring was seen in all the three generations but was more commonly seen in F0 and F1 generation.

The increase in the lifestyle-related diseases of obesity, hypertension, and metabolic disturbances is of concern and needs to be tackled at multiple levels beginning from early childhood.

**Tables 6.1.1:**
*Summary of descriptive variables for the three generations among age group 4-12 years of the NDBC*

| Variables | F2 Generation (N=229) Age 4–12 Years | | F1 Generation | | F0 Generation | | |
| | N | Mean ± SD | N | F1 Parent (Mean ± SD) | N | Grandfather (Mean ± SD) | Grandmother (Mean ± SD) |
| --- | --- | --- | --- | --- | --- | --- | --- |
| Age (years) | 228 | 8.6 ± 2.2 | | | | | |
| Weight (kg) | 221 | 29.9 ± 11.6 | 219 | 74.0 ± 13.5 | 182 | 68.9 ± 12.2 | 65.6 ± 12.5 |
| Height (cm) | 222 | 129.7 ± 14.9 | 219 | 165.4 ± 9.0 | 182 | 163.9 ± 5.9 | 150.1 ± 6.8 |
| Systolic Blood Pressure (mmHg) | 210 | 102.7 ± 9.5 | 219 | 128.7 ± 17.5 | 182 | 149.7 ± 26.2 | 146.4 ± 22.9 |
| Diastolic Blood Pressure (mmHg) | 210 | 64.3 ± 8.5 | 219 | 83.4 ± 12.1 | 182 | 82.4 ± 12.1 | 82.0 ± 10.1 |
| Pulse Rate (per min) | 210 | 92.9 ± 13.3 | 217 | 83.7 ± 9.6 | 182 | 76.9 ± 11.0 | 81.20 ± 10.3 |
| Plasma Fasting Glucose (mg/dL) | 155 | 83.8 ± 10.3 | 193 | 101.9 ± 41.8 | 127 | 117.9 ± 45.0 | 112.6 ± 45.9 |
| Total Cholesterol (mg/dL) | 157 | 164.8 ± 31.9 | 193 | 199.8 ± 40.4 | 130 | 183.3 ± 47.1 | 202.4 ± 44.3 |
| HDL Cholesterol (mg/dL) | 157 | 51.4 ± 10.4 | 193 | 47.0 ± 11.7 | 130 | 46.7 ± 11.9 | 52.0 ± 12.3 |
| LDL Cholesterol (mg/dL) | 93 | 89.4 ± 21.8 | 124 | 123.1 ± 30.7 | 104 | 113.5 ± 39.1 | 122.3 ± 41.2 |
| Triglycerides (mg/dL) | 157 | 90.0 ± 36.1 | 193 | 151.4 ± 78.1 | 130 | 122.6 ± 62.3 | 144.2 ± 62.9 |
| Haemoglobin (g/dL) | 89 | 11.7 ± 1.5 | 171 | 12.7 ± 1.9 | 102 | 12.3 ± 1.9 | 11.2 ± 1.65 |

**Source:** Author.

**Table 6.1.2:**
*Summary of descriptive variables for the three generations among age group >12 years of the NDBC*

| Variables | F2 Generation (N=122) Age >12 Years | | F1 Generation | | F0 Generation | | | |
| | N | Mean±SD | N | F1 Parent (Mean±SD) | N | Grandfather (Mean±SD) | N | Grandmother (Mean±SD) |
|---|---|---|---|---|---|---|---|---|
| Age (years) | 121 | 14.6±1.96 | | | | | | |
| Weight (kg) | 121 | 51.0±13.9 | 115 | 72.8±14.0 | 63 | 65.3±12.3 | 100 | 65.4±13.3 |
| Height (cm) | 121 | 157.3±9.0 | 115 | 162.8±9.0 | 64 | 162.2±5.4 | 100 | 150.0±5.6 |
| Systolic Blood Pressure (mmHg) | 120 | 106.6±11.1 | 114 | 124.3±14.4 | 63 | 142.9±21.5 | 99 | 143.7±19.6 |
| Diastolic Blood Pressure (mmHg) | 120 | 66.4±8.4 | 114 | 81.7±10.8 | 63 | 78.5±10.6 | 99 | 81.4±10.1 |
| Pulse Rate (per min) | 120 | 83.9±10.4 | 114 | 83.3±9.2 | 63 | 76.7±13.1 | 99 | 80.8±11.0 |
| Plasma Fasting Glucose (mg/dL) | 105 | 83.4±9.7 | 109 | 97.1±16.9 | 43 | 116.0±39.0 | 77 | 109.3±36.2 |
| Total Cholesterol (mg/dL) | 106 | 156.0±28.3 | 109 | 201.6±41.6 | 43 | 185.5±40.1 | 77 | 204.5±43.1 |
| HDL Cholesterol (mg/dL) | 106 | 47.9±10.9 | 109 | 47.5±10.7 | 43 | 46.6±12.7 | 77 | 50.3±11.0 |
| LDL Cholesterol (mg/dL) | 76 | 89.6±22.3 | 67 | 130.7±35.1 | 37 | 112.7±34.0 | 62 | 126.1±37.1 |
| Triglycerides (mg/dL) | 106 | 95.2±34.8 | 109 | 147.5±82.9 | 43 | 130.6±75.8 | 77 | 148.3±62.5 |
| Haemoglobin (g/dL) | 75 | 12.1±1.9 | 101 | 12.1±1.8 | 37 | 12.6±2.1 | 59 | 11.5±1.4 |

*Source:* Author.

# 2

# The Third Generation

At the last follow-up of the family cohort, we had 3,572 children of F2 generation. It has not been possible to investigate all of these children in the manner as their parents were investigated. This has been largely due to our focus on the life cycle of the NDBC and due to constraints of finance and other resources. However, these children who form the third generation of the NDBC whenever accompanied by their parents to the field clinics, were enrolled on a pretested paediatric pro forma, which provided details about their general medical history, perinatal and birth history, physical examination, feeding, growth and development, and others. Then, as per interest or concern, certain emerging specific problems of public health importance were also investigated. The data on the children is, therefore, not as continuous or age specific as for F1. The information on them and the studies were performed and collected randomly.

## General Profile

The mean birth weight of the F2 children was 2,817.2 g. The LBW prevalence was 18.0%. As mentioned earlier, the mean birth weight was slightly lower than F1, but the LBW prevalence had decreased substantially. Menarche was recorded to occur from the age of 10 years, but 1/3rd or 28.3% had it at 13 years and 35% at 14 years. In 23.3%, menarche occurred between 15 and 19 years of age. In comparison, in the generation of the parents, the median and interquartile range for age of menarche in F1 was 14.0 and 10–19 years respectively. The third or the F2 children generation of the NDBC were investigated for selective disorders. These included the cardiovascular risk factors, sleep disorders, behaviour disorders, and hand grip studies. Over 1,000 children varying from 4–19 years were studied for these disorders at different points of time. A brief description of these studies is provided below.

1. **Cardiovascular Risk Factors in Adolescent Children**
   Cardiovascular risk factors were investigated in over 250 adolescent children (F2 generation) of 10–18 years of age. The risk factors investigated included overweight/obesity, central obesity, pre-hypertension and hypertension, impaired fasting blood glucose level, and dyslipidaemia. An attempt was also made to relate these to the maternal height and sitting height.

   Prevalence of overweight was almost 25%, and 5.3% of children were obese. Central obesity was recorded in 1/5th or 22.4% of the children. Pre-hypertension was more frequent in girls (18.4%) as compared to boys (10.4%). Hypertension was noted in 7.7%; it was almost three times (12.2%) as common in girls as compared to boys (4.4%). Impaired fasting glucose concentration was found in 10%, hyper-triglyceridemia in 10.2%, and low HDL prevalence in 23.5% of adolescents (Figure 6.2.1).

   The study did not find any association between height and sitting height of the mother with cardiovascular risk factors. This may have been due to relatively smaller sample size.

   The high prevalence of the cardiovascular risk factors was a disconcerting finding, which pointed to the need of close monitoring of health especially in children with overweight and obesity, regular check on blood pressure, and with any indication, investigation for a full profile of cardiometabolic risk markers.

2. **Sleep Patterns and Factors Influencing them in Children of NDBC**
   Sleep disorders and sleep-related morbidities are becoming an active area of interest for clinicians and researchers in children. In India, its relevance is now being increasingly realized in relation to a child's behaviour, performance, and cardiometabolic disorders. We studied the problem in over 250 children from 4–18 years. The children were divided into two groups of 4–12 years

**Figure 6.2.1:**
*Cardiovascular risk factors in F2 adolescences*

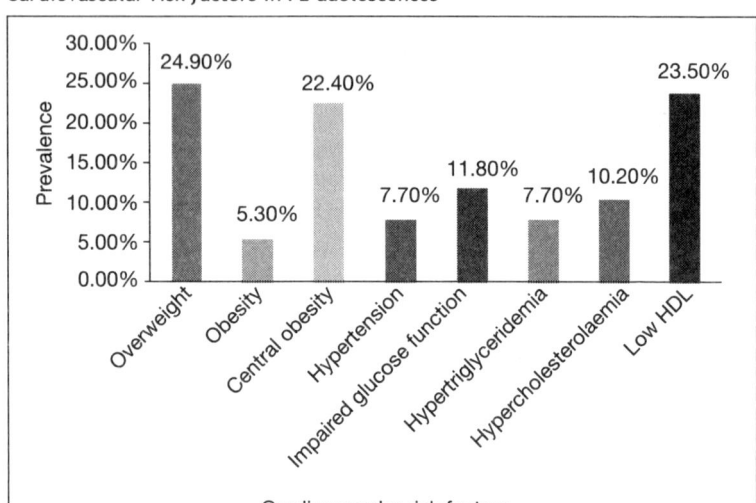

*Source:* Author.

and 12–18 years. The study aimed to elicit sleep patterns sleep problems and its association with body weight and body growth. Two distinct groups of problems became apparent. The first related to the sleep patterns and the prevalence of sleep problem, and the second the association between overweight/obesity and BMI with sleep behaviour of the children.

The children fell off to sleep easily and had no problem in this habit of sleep. The sleep duration was recorded to be longer on weekend in all the children. Similarly, the bed time and wake up time was delayed during weekends. This may be related to the weekend being a school holiday. Older children slept more on weekends as their sleep time was later than younger children. The children felt the best in evening time. TV watching increased over weekends and this could contribute to late sleeping and getting up time, especially in older children.

Parasomnias comprising a group of symptoms such as grinding of teeth, nightmares, enuresis, and sleep walking were more common in younger children. Both the group of children fell asleep easily in day time. This happened while sitting, going in car, reading, watching television, etc. Co-sleeping was common in the younger children who often slept with parents or grandparents, siblings, or other relatives.

Snoring was seen in both groups. It was commonly associated with overweight and obesity in the subjects. Overweight and obesity was more common in older children. It had a suggestion of association with shorter sleep duration.

3. **Behavioural Problems and their Association with School Performance**

   Increasing behaviour problems in schoolgoing children are emerging concerns, and are being increasingly recognized as a cause influencing scholastic performance in them.

   F2 generation were assessed by a child behaviour checklist (CBCL) and children global assessment scale (CGAS) for prevalence of severity of behaviour disturbance. These were then related to their school performances by using grades and other indicators of performance as school pro forma. The school performance was then classified into high achievers (grade A1, A2), scholastically average (B1, B2, and C1), and scholastically low (C2 and below).

   Surprisingly, 48%, or roughly every other child showed some behaviour problem. Prevalence of behavioural problems based on total CBCL score and CGAS (using impairment criteria < 70) was 15.5%. Most of the children with behaviour problems were high achievers with A1 and A2 grades, with 10% being low achieves (C2 grades) and remaining as average (B1 and C1 grades).

   Interestingly, low maternal education, long TV watching hours, and time spent on computer was associated with behavioural problems. The school performance was significantly affected by behaviour problems. School absenteeism was also associated with behaviour problems. Parental involvement improved school performance and was even better than those who took tuitions.

   The pattern of specific behaviour problems included withdrawn/depression (2.0%), anxious (2.0%), enuresis (10.0%), and aggressive defiant disorder and delinquent behaviour (2.5% each). Attention deficit hyperactive disorder was seen in only 1.5% and isolated phobia in 5%. Significantly, most children with behaviour problems had poor school performance.

4. **Hand Grip Strength and its Relationship to Birth Weight and Adult Health**

   Hand grip is most commonly used for hand shake and other day-to-day activities, is the result of forceful reflex on of all finger joints with the maximum voluntary force that a subject is able to exert under normal bio-kinetic condition. It is commonly used to assess the upper body strength, which is influenced by several factors. It is influenced by in-utero development, and birth weight in a way is a reflection of this. The hand grip strength has been found to be related to health outcomes in adults and geriatric population. Therefore, there is a search to relate hand grip as an early indicator in childhood for later adult outcomes such as metabolic syndrome and CAD.

F2 adolescent children were investigated to measure their muscle strength and its relationship to birth weight, and to relate the muscle strength with body anthropometric measurements and body composition. This was done to evaluate if any association exists between hand grip strength and metabolic syndrome or any of its components including adiposity, blood pressure, glucose imbalance, or lipid profile.

The F2 children varied between 10 and 19 years of age. The measurements, using standard techniques, included handgrip strength, anthropometric and body composition measurements of body weight, height, mid arm, waist, and hip circumferences, and skin fold thickness from several sites such as triceps, biceps, sub-scapular, and supra iliac fold. Blood pressure and biochemical parameters as described earlier were also measured.

Two hundred and ninety children were measured with almost equal number of boys and girls. As expected, the boys at all ages had greater anthropometric measurements. In simple as well as in age- and gender-adjusted analysis, a significant association existed between grip strength and anthropometric and body composition variable of metabolic syndrome such as BMI, fat mass, lean mass, and systolic and diastolic blood pressures. However, waist to hip ratio was not associated with grip strength in crude as well as in adjusted (age, gender, weight, and height) analysis. No significant association was found between the biochemical variables (fasting plasma glucose, cholesterol, HDL, LDL, and triglyceride level) of metabolic syndrome with grip strength.

In the present study results, firm conclusions could not be drawn and further studies on a larger sample may be required to establish usefulness of hand grip as a screening tool for determining risk of cardiometabolic disorders in children.

# PART 7

# Community Expectation and Challenges

# 1

# Attrition or Loss to Follow-Up

The NDBC has been a longitudinal study, which is now in its fifth decade. It was, therefore, expected to lose cohort subjects over this long period. This has been the experience of most of the longitudinal cohort studies. The NDBC has been conducted in eight phases with gaps of 3–8 years between the different phases. At the beginning of each phase, a census was done to assess the attrition or loss of cohort in the intervening period and the number of cohorts likely to be available for conducting the new studies.

We have used the following terms to describe various kinds of loss to follow-up during the cohort follow-up from 1969 to 2017.

1. **Shifted or Moved Out or Moved In Cases**
   This nomenclature has been used for the families or individuals who moved out of the area by reasons of transfers, starting new ventures, immigration, or for unknown reasons. A 'moved out' report was made, and an attempt was made to ascertain the new address and also the reasons for the shift.

2. **Permanent Loss Cases**
   In most cases, the fact of moving out was known only after the 'move' and without the subject leaving any forwarding address to other places. An effort was made to trace the family's new address by sending a 'tracer'. If the new address was not found nor any information became available, it was categorized as permanent loss.

3. **Temporary Loss**

   This term was used when the cohort subjects could not be contacted due to any of the following reasons but their whereabouts and contact details were available.

   a. Residing outside NCR (National Capital Region) and could not come for the follow-up.
   b. Residing outside the country.
   c. Either not came or not included for follow-up due to unavoidable reasons such as chronic illness, pregnancy, or other reason.
   d. In some cohorts, there was genuine fear of a blood test or its result. They were almost paranoid about it.
   e. Some cohorts simply expressed their total inability to come to the clinics on the clinic days due to prior commitments.

4. **Reluctant**

   Those cohorts who initially showed their willingness to attend clinic on a project personal visit to them, but never kept their appointments for the follow-ups and were perpetually giving varied reasons for not attending clinics.

5. **Refusal**

   This included those cohorts who were not willing to continue their follow-ups for any reason and were not willing to participate in further studies.

6. **Expired**

   Some cohorts passed away during the follow-ups and these were categorized as expired.

## Attrition in Different Phases of NDBC

The project was established in 1969–73 with 8,181 cohorts in Phase I. At the end of Phase I, 457 cohorts had died. The next census was done at the beginning of Phase II in 1974 and we had 7,724 surviving cohorts. Of the 7,724 cohorts, we could trace 7,119, losing another 605 (8.4%) children between Phases I and the end of Phase II in December 1980. The next census was at the beginning of Phase III and was done during 1983–87. Of the 7,119 subjects at the end of Phase II, we could trace only 4,705, losing a whopping 2,414 (33.3%) of cohorts between Phases II and III. This was shocking but happened due to large-scale demolitions which were done by the Municipal Corporation of New Delhi, and the lost cohort resettled elsewhere without leaving a forwarding address. The next round of census was done in Phase IV in 1988–90. We located 4,104 cohorts, losing 601 (12.7%) of the cohorts. This was a selective phase to identify and follow-up only those cohorts who were likely to reach the age of 20 years by 1990. Thus, of the 3,337 cohorts that we had enrolled, 1,030 were selected for further follow-up. Of these 1,030, we could not locate 194 children and, hence, included only 836 children for completion of adult studies. Thus, the NDBC had lost 4,844 (59.2%) of the cohorts between its foundation in 1969–73 to the end of childhood phase in 1991.

The fifth round of census was done in 1998–2003 when the project was being revived after 8 years. At this time, significant changes had occurred in the administrative set up as the writer had left his employment at Safdarjung Hospital and shifted to a private hospital and a private paediatric consultancy. A new team had to be appointed and the research office had to be shifted to a rented accommodation. The new appointees were not as skilled or trained as the previous team of field workers and had to be trained in the task of retracing, which included posting letters, telephone calls, and visit to the field area and completing a pro forma. We were fortunate to employ a senior anthropologist (Ms Verma) who was familiar with the fieldwork and field area and knew the cohorts personally. This helped in tracking. and we were able to track 2,584 of the 3,337 cohorts who were available at the end of the Phase IV and thus lost 753 (22.5%). This was expected as the cohort had grown as young adults and finished their education. Most of them were employed; many of them had married and had their own families and children and had moved out of their from their parent's house to other parts of city or elsewhere.

Phase VI of census was from 2003–06 when a new project was being initiated by the NDBC group. At this time, we tracked 1,759 of 2,584 cohorts available at the end of the last phase. We thus lost 825 (31.9%). This was not expected, but may be due to the cohorts leaving their parental house to establish themselves or finding new jobs, which required a shift of residence.

Phase VII of the project was conducted between the years 2006 and 2009. We lost 377 cohorts and were left with 1,382. This seems to be an underestimate and may be due to change of staff or recording error.

The seventh phase follow-up was started in September 2015 as a routine to keep track of the cohort. We were now working from a redrawn list of 3,352 cohorts and we have been able to track 2,105 of these cohorts. This phase has actually shown an increase from the last tracing and may due to the vigorous effort of the staff to try to reach every cohort till repeated efforts to trace failed (Table 7.1.1).

**Table 7.1.1:**
*Attrition in various phases of the NDBC study*

| Phases | Project | Duration of Project | Number of Cohort at Beginning of the Phase | Cohorts Lost to Follow-Up | Number of Cohorts | Cohort at the End of the Phase |
|---|---|---|---|---|---|---|
| Phase I | Longitudinal study of the survival and outcome of a birth cohort | April 1969 to 31 July 1973 | 8,181 | 1,062 | 457 (deaths) | 605 |
| Between Phase I and II | | | | 2,414 | | |
| Phase II | Longitudinal study of the survival and outcome of a birth cohort | May 1974 to December, 1980 | 4,705 | 601 | Break up not available | — |
| Between Phase II and III | | | | 767 | Break up not available | — |
| Phase III | Longitudinal study of the survival and outcome of a birth cohort | July 1983 to December 1987 | 3,337 | 493 | Break up not available | — |
| Phase IV | Longitudinal study of the survival and outcome of a birth cohort from 17 to 20 yrs of age | 1 January 1988 to 13 July 1991 | 2,844/1,092* children were selected in the beginning for the study. | 256 | | |
| Phase V | Maternal Nutrition, foetal growth, and coronary risk factor in young adults | November 1998 to December 2003 | 3,419* (Project was revived after 8 years) | 835 | | 2,584 |

| Phase | Topic | Date | Follow-up details | | Loss details | Total |
|---|---|---|---|---|---|---|
| Phase VI | Relationship of growth in infancy and childhood to adult endothelial function and body composition: The New Delhi Birth Cohort | March 2006 to June 2009 | 2,584/1,526* (Selective follow-up of those who attained clinic in Phase V) | 377 | | |
| Phase VII | Trans-generational sleep Patterns, co-morbidities and body composition in 'The New Delhi Birth Cohort' | April 2009 to May 2011 | Selective follow-up* (All three generation alive (trio) available = 970 (approx.) | 1,117 | 772 (cases lost due to death) + 898 (could not be located) + 142 (refusal) | 2,221 |
| Phase VIII | 1. Genetic determinants of birth weight and growth trajectory and influence of parental genotype on these anthropometric indicators. 2. Relationship of birth size, infant and childhood growth on telomere length in adulthood. | 2012 to 2015 | Selective follow-up* (All three generation alive (trio) available = 970 (approx.) of list taken 3,337 | 1,189 | 772 (cases lost due to death) + 914 (could not be located) + 198 (refusal) | 2,148 |

*Source:* Author.
*Note:* * Follow-up of only those cohorts who were likely to reach the age of 20 years by 1990.

The variable numbers at the beginning or at the end of the census is not surprising. It happened to us all the time as we came across some lead or some news of a cohort from a neighbour, relative, a friend, or another cohort and then tried to track them.

## Factors Contributing to Loss of Cohorts

There have been many reasons for the losses, which include deaths that are natural in a population, shifting of the population without leaving an address to other parts of the city, or migrating from the city of Delhi to other parts of India or even other countries. We analyzed selective factors to see if the loss to follow-up was uniformly spread or was selective in nature.

Tracking the cohorts is a very difficult task. It is not customary nor in our nature to leave forwarding address when changing accommodation. Tenancy is a major problem in Delhi due to the crunch of accommodation, demands, and tenancy laws. The lease for rental is usually for 11 months and the tenant, and in this case the cohorts, may be required to change their accommodation several times.

We tried to leave a stamped envelope with our address and telephone number. But the cohorts very rarely informed either by post or telephone. We would ask the neighbours for the cohort but the help was hardly forthcoming. We even tried to find through the postman of the area and post office but this too was not successful.

The other difficulties in tracking were haphazard numbering and, therefore, at times a new appointee could not locate the house and would report it as loss to follow-up. Many a times the houses were locked or the parents had gone on vacation or holiday, especially during summer and winter school breaks and vacations. Extreme weather conditions also contributed to reporting of loss of cohort as we felt the effort was not enough by the team.

A peculiar social problem was the parent's refusal to give the address of their married female daughter. It made them afraid that a long follow-up may be considered as a social stigma by the in-laws or misunderstood as a medical history not told to them.

An analysis for causes of loss to follow-up showed the maximum losses to occur with the type of residence of cohorts. It was the highest residents of jhuggis and single-room rental dwellers, especially in the initial Phases II and III.

A major cause of loss to follow-up of the cohorts was demolition of unauthorized housing or localities. At the time of emergency in the country, several colonies which were considered unauthorized were demolished. Several hundred cohorts used to live in these colonies.

Income of parents seemed to influence the loss to follow-up. Cohorts earning low income or those earning high incomes were the one to be most affected by the loss to follow-up. It is possible that both strata of the extremes of income required changing their residence more frequently, albeit for different reasons.

Educational status also affected cohort loss to follow-up. Illiterates seemed to be the one who were lost in larger numbers than educated. Religion of the cohort was another factor related to loss to follow-up. For some reason, more Muslims were lost to follow-up than from other religions.

Subjects born LBW were also lost in larger numbers. It is possible that some of them may have died or it is possible that LBW being associated with multiple causes, sequelae, and other causes may have also contributed to the loss to follow-up.

# 2

## Cohort Participation

### Introduction

At a time when there is growing acceptance and understanding of the value of longitudinal research, it has become increasingly difficult to recruit and, more importantly, retain participants in a longitudinal study. It is one of the few longitudinal birth cohort studies which have been followed by one of the founders and his colleagues from preconception of the cohorts to conception, birth, and infancy and through different periods of childhood to adulthood. During this period, it has evolved from a single generation cohort to a four-generation family cohort. All longitudinal studies lose participants over the years due to a variety of reasons. However, little has been researched into the reasons as to why respondents have remained or not remained in a study and what strategies could be developed or adopted to improve retention. It would, therefore, be interesting and useful to know from the NDBC experience as to what prompted the subjects to continue participation in the study for almost half a century without any medical, financial, or similar incentives.

The participation of the subjects was totally voluntary. They were not offered any incentives or compensation in cash or kind for their time or transport for attending field clinics. They welcomed the field staff in their home and there is not a single instance of any kind of dispute, fight, or argument, even when a cohort refused to participate.

It was the mothers (FO generation) who had enrolled in the field follow-up as an ever-married, non-pregnant woman for the study, and then as mothers and guardians of their offspring through childhood to adulthood. Once cohort members became independent young adults, it became solely their decision to remain a part of the study. In due course of time, their children (F2) had been enrolled, and as they grew and became adult, some of them married and had children and they too became part of the NDBC cohort family. The whole of the NDBC cohort families willingly participated in numerous and different clinics and studies.

## Trust of the Cohorts

One of the most frequently asked question has been as to how we have been able to continue and sustain the cohort and the research in a low middle-income country like India. The question seekers have wondered as to how it has been possible without offering any kind of compensation to cohorts. How did the cohorts accept that we did not offer any medical advice and intervention? Truly, we do not know have the answer to these questions. But, what we firmly believe is that it was the implicit trust between the cohorts and their families and the founders and the research team which kept us together and allowed the NDBC and its studies and investigations to flourish. In the last five decades, the cohorts have never questioned our intentions or objectives. They have firmly believed that whatever we are doing is for their good, is good for the community and for the research, and a good cause. They also felt confident that we will put the results of the research to good use for mankind and will never abuse or misuse them. What surprised us was their willingness to allow us numerous blood tests, computed tomography (CT) scans, DEXA scans, electrocardiogram (ECG), echocardiographies (ECHO), cognitive and psychological, and a variety of other clinical tests. Their understanding and cooperation was truly amazing and very satisfying, which encouraged us to continue the study despite many road blocks and difficulties.

The other striking reason came from the cohort themselves. They felt very happy and proud to be a participant in this unique study. They felt it like a personal fulfilment and satisfaction. Some even felt it was their duty and obligation to participate. Another feature which was noted was the increasing interest and questions, which they began to ask as the study progressed. This showed their interest and involvement. Some felt it was a journey of a lifetime for them, and this in some way evoked a sense of commitment in them to be part of the NDBC story.

The cohorts also remembered many other pleasant experiences. They remembered that from the time they were born we visited them at specific age till they were adults of 20 years of age. They recounted the stories the research team told them about the body measurements, equipment, their increase in body weight, and the adolescence queries and anxieties. In brief, they considered the research as their own and the research team as their families.

## Convenience of Cohort

From the inception of the study, we had been extremely particular regarding the convenience of cohorts and maintaining the privacy and confidentiality of the information they provided. We visited their homes for data collection only by prior appointment after seeking the time most convenient to them. The collection of the entire data in the childhood phase was home based. In the adult phase, the clinics had to be conducted in the field. We organized clinics in different areas within a certain radius of their home so that it was easier and convenient for them. We used gentle telephone or personal reminders if they missed appointments and clinic visits and never complained even if several appointments were missed. We ensured collection of maximum information at each visit to minimize their visits or interaction with the research team. This was most appreciated and ensured their participation.

## Distribution and Interpretation of Reports

All efforts were made to ensure that the results of the anthropometry and other tests were communicated to them in writing. Original signed reports of all the tests were delivered to them at home or, in case of a very long distance, sent by post. This assured the continued co-operation of the cohort and they returned for their follow-up time and again.

# Interactive Meetings with Cohorts

Interactive meetings were organized with the cohorts as a kind of informal get together. In these meetings, the cohorts were invited to come and interact with foreign and Indian investigators. All the investigators used to share their expertise and experience and explain the need to do these studies. The cohorts were encouraged to speak and ask questions and share feelings and impressions about the project and staff. This created a friendly atmosphere and feelings that helped run the project.

## Challenges to Cohort's Participation

1. **Participants Fatigue**
   The NDBC is a longitudinal study and had been running for many years. We were visiting or calling them over a period again and again, asking repetitive or long questions, and interviewing them for long periods, which required waiting in the clinics. This was likely to result in fatigue or a feeling that enough is enough. We scrupulously and consciously avoided these. We kept the number of visits of the staff, telephone calls, or visits to the clinic to the barest minimum. An effort was made to utilize the clinic visit to the utmost utility. We always apologized for the inconvenience and explained each time the need for a visit, or a call, or an appointment.

2. **Participants' Consent and Assents**
   At the beginning of the project and through the childhood phase, we used to obtain verbal consent. In the adult phase, all consents were written and signed with a participant information sheet. This made it necessary for the staff to explain the reason for the visit, the study, tests, and other aspects. Each visit of the cohort enhanced their knowledge about the objectives and methods of the study. This again helped in better return visits and compliance.

3. **Confidentiality**
   The cohorts were concerned about confidentiality of their illness, disease, and tests results. We made sure that all the tests results and reports were given to the cohorts personally or delivered at home. All reports were discussed in private in one-to-one consultations.

In the beginning of Phase I in 1969–73, we had to face the confidentiality issue. All the cohorts were women. They were sensitive about their menstrual period, missed periods, and about their conception. This was one of the major challenges of winning trust as we had just begun the project. We had designed the pro forma in such a way that the information till a pregnancy follow-up began remained confidential with data managers and supervisors.

4. **Sharing Problems**

   As a policy, we had decided to communicate directly with the cohorts for any change of programme or delay in analysis of a report or a false or wrong report. We were frank about it and discussed openly and shared these with them. This increased confidence and trust of the cohort.

## Cohort Indifference and Problems

1. **Refusal**–In spite of our best efforts, we lost confidence or trust of the cohort and they became a reluctant participant to the study. They refused because of their own accord or because of parents or husbands.

2. **Indifference**–The cohorts developed fatigue or indifference due to repeated visits. Some of them simply failed to appreciate the relevance of the study and considered it a burden to find time to attend the clinic.

3. **Family planning worker**–In the initial phase, the community thought us to be family planning workers. They simply did not want to meet them and refused to see or interact with the workers. The year 1970 was the era of family planning and, in particular, of sterilization and promotion of Copper T tube.

4. **Long clinic hours and waiting**–At times, the clinic became overcrowded, or the entire staff was not in attendance, or we had some other logistic issue. At such times, a cohort had to wait on an average for 2½ hours and, hence, a longer stay made a cohort reluctant to attend in the future.

5. **Reports**–We normally tried to deliver all the reports within 3 weeks' time as this interval was required by us for checking the reports, making their entry, and typing for delivery. A delay irritated the cohort and made him say that the reports come so late

that they are not worth it. We tried our best to explain but many a time we did not succeed.

6.  **Expectations**–For many cohorts we fell below their expectations. Their usual question being what they will get from participation as we did not offer any rewards, incentives, or medical intervention. As we came from large and renowned institutions they wanted some favours or their medical needs to be addressed. It was a difficult proposal because of the crowds and rush in government hospitals and cost in private hospitals.

7.  **Communications**–At times they were serious but avoidable communication misunderstandings. Our messages were not understood or were misunderstood. We did not have mobile phone, emails, and landline phones were scarce. We had to communicate by personal contact and sometimes there were failures.

8.  **Ethical issues**–In the adult phase, a written informed consent was mandatory. The NDBC sometime had several projects which required multiple consents. This bothered the cohorts and sometimes they refused one or the other consent.

9.  **Environment**–The clinics were held in temples, gurudwaras (Sikh temples), schools and private homes, or other rented accommodations. Sometimes these were not very clean, hygienic, open, and well ventilated. They were at times too hot or cold due to inadequate cooling or warming facilities. This caused discomfort, and to be in the same environment for 2–3 hours caused some inconvenience.

10. **Faith, beliefs, and superstition**–This was a major problem when the cohort was being established. There were myths and beliefs about pregnancy becoming known, or a child to be weighed, or to be seen by a stranger or even examined by a doctor. This used to be quite a difficult part to convince them that these are myths but nothing could be done due to the firm belief of the community.

## Strategies to Enhance Cohorts' Participation

1.  One of them was the dissemination about health information. We tried to personally explain about the diseases, distribute pamphlets, or tried to hold meeting with the cohorts to share our experiences. We asked Indian and foreign investigators to attend these

social kind of get-togethers and meetings and requested them to share their experiences. The response was variable and not always encouraging.

2. We did the health check-up of the family or friends whom they brought with them during the field clinic. We did not refuse, but also did not particularly encourage this as it involved tests with costs.

3. We provided consultations to their family and relatives free of any charge as this was acceptable in research protocols. They wanted referrals to known specialists and hospitals, which were provided. This helped in enhancing our reputation as a friendly team.

4. We were very particular in keeping track of our outstation cohorts who lived away from Delhi and came periodically to visit their families. We tried to call or email them for clinic assessment during their visit by staying in touch.

5. We tried to organise clinics at a suitable neighbourhood venue and on days when there was a possibility of a large turnout. These were public holidays or children vacations or festival periods.

6. We organized special clinics at home for physically challenged or elderly F0 parents of the cohort.

7. Mop-up clinics: In spite of all these efforts, cohorts missed an appointment or a field clinic with one excuse or another. To ensure their continued participation, we used to organize mop-up clinics in the same area near their residence. This helped increase the number of follow-up and maintained the longitudinal nature of the study.

# PART 8

# Implications and Impact

# Introduction

The NDBC in its journey of five decades has accumulated considerable experience in establishing and successfully running a longitudinal study in a country like India. It has, therefore, many experiences and results of its research which have implications and impact in planning, conducting, collaborating, and prioritizing for implementation and adoption in national public health policies in the health delivery system for children and adults.

# 1

# Public Health and Policies

1. **Public Health**
   The selection of the study area and population required considerable thinking, effort, and discussion amongst investigators. We had several constrains and conditions for the launching of this study. The study had to be population-based, providing a spectrum of demographic profile of the family, and the women had to be followed from pre-pregnant state to pregnancy and birth of the child. The gestational age and birth weight of the newborn had to be correctly known and recorded. The area had to be physically defined and demarcated. It was a typical urban, large, metro, mixed population representing all section of the society in the social, cultural, education, environment, and income profile of an urban community.

   The selection of the study area and population were fully justified by the NDBC studies to have still remained relevant and of contemporary interest contributing constantly to research and public health issues.

   The NDBC project was primarily established to find the outcome, survival, and sequelae of LBW children by a prospective cohort study. As the study got extended with new grants every three to four years, its objectives were modified as per available data and in the context of current appropriate research needs. In the first two decades, the NDBC made several observations on maternal and child health and collected data but were mainly focused on longitudinal growth of cohort children with the sole objective of establishing norms for growth of urban Indian children from birth to 20 years of age.

In the 1990s, the objectives were redefined to test Barker's hypothesis of foetal origin of adult diseases. In further active collaboration, the NDBC with similar cohorts from four other low middle-income countries studied extensively the childhood growth, body composition, BMI, and its association with adult diseases such as diabetes, metabolic syndrome, cardiovascular disorders, and others. It also investigated the association between body growth and human capital development and its influence on birth weight of the next progeny. The NDBC expanded its studies to genes associated with diabetes, body growth, and lipid disturbances.

In its five decades of existence, the NDBC has now evolved into a family cohort with its four generations. We have studied the intergeneration and trans-generation influences on diseases and explored with pilot studies selective areas for research in F2 generation or children of the cohorts.

The ever-continuing investigation and collaboration of the NDBC demonstrates that such studies are possible, can be dynamic and flexible to modify objectives with time and resources, and remain relevant and interesting even today. In a sense, the decades of research exemplifies the need and necessity of long-term cohort studies and investment in resources for such studies in public health.

2. **Population Explosion and Family Welfare**

The NDBC focused on the problem of population explosion and high fertility prevalence at that time. The government had identified fertility control and family planning as one of the foremost problems and adopted it as a national programme. The findings confirmed high total fertility rate in the urban community and identified teenage marriage, birth of the first child with a short period of consummation of marriage, education and socio-economic indicator, child mortality and pregnancy wastage, and less than two year interval between successive births as major contributors to the problem of high fertility rate and not-so-successful family planning programme. Educating the women, enforcement of Sharda Act which prohibited teenage marriage, and public awareness programmes emerged as a meaningful national measure for control of population. One of the major deterrents to adoption of family planning was the child mortality experience by the family. This indicated the need to improve child survival as the key to limit family in a positive constructive way. The NDBC along with findings and experience of their researches may have led to the formulation and adoption of child survival as a national policy.

3. **Pregnancy Outcome**

The NDBC studies were done in a population with relatively better socio-economic conditions and education located in an area with easy access to facility and institution-based health care. But despite this, the antenatal care and delivery practices showed poor utilization and awareness. The antenatal registration was good, but the visit for antenatal care in the three trimesters was dismal. The community largely knew its preferences and options, and as many as 40% opted for domiciliary or home delivery. The findings offered a clear message for improving public awareness on benefits of proper and regular antenatal care and advantages of institution-based deliveries. It indicated the need for health education programmes on improved and better outcome of pregnancy with appropriate and timely antenatal visits and utilization of health care facilities.

# 2

# The NDBC Research

1. **Cohort Research**

   The NDBC is now a depository of research with lessons relevant for all times in different kinds and natures of long-term research. It describes the development of different hypothesis, study design, methodologies, protocol development, longitudinal data collection and storage, and use of constantly changing methodologies for analytical techniques, interpretation of study results, and their applications.

   The choice of study design as a cohort study in an urban population on a subject like LBW, which was not only a burning problem then but continues to remain of public health interest, emphasizes the need for clarity in defining immediate and long-term objectives and their expected outcome at the initial planning stage and with passage of time and progress of the study.

   The NDBC faced numerous challenges from financial support to developing projects, seeking collaboration, and finding suitable human and technical resources for keeping the study meaningful. But the successful running of this cohort study in its fifth decade from a time when research of such nature was unthinkable, resources in terms of finance, trained manpower, and tools for investigation, and data analysis not readily available indicates that it is a possible to initiate and undertake research of such nature in difficult circumstances with determination, commitment, and foresight.

   The rapport of the research team with cohorts for almost 50 years highlights the need of a constant interaction with the community, understanding their needs and expectations, and responding satisfactorily to their concerns. The cohort participation was totally voluntary. They were not compensated for their time or travel to the field clinics. It showed that it is possible to undertake such projects without monetary incentives but by a skilful, persuasive interaction and explanation to community.

The extensive collaborations at national and international level underlines the willingness and open-minded approach to acceptance of challenging research and spirit of sharing data, experience, and trust with like-minded researchers. This is perhaps the key to be a part of successful collaborative research.

2. **Intrauterine Growth of Cohort**

The foetal growth curves of the NDBC pointed that these are comparable to other population curves till 34 weeks of pregnancy, but the growth decelerated or flattened thereafter. It's hard to explain, but something happens at this time of pregnancy which needs to be investigated and studied.

The other pertinent question in this regard is to whether consider Indian foetal growth curves as standards or to accept the WHO International INTERGROWTH-21 foetal curves as foetal growth standards. This is a tricky question as Indian researchers and others from developing countries had argued and questioned the acceptance of definition of LBW on the basis of prevalence, morbidity, and mortality. The NDBC data has shown that thin children who become overweight or obese are prone to adult chronic metabolic and heart diseases. Trans-generation studies have shown that the growth of the children is significantly improving and has shown a positive change. Extending this logic or reasoning, if we chase the international growth curves and try to increase the growth of the foetus beyond its potential, we do not know whether we will push the child to an advantage or to an adverse outcome in later life. These are areas of concern and debatable issues which emerge from this cohort study.

3. **Low Birth Weight**

The NDBC was established to investigate the problem of LBW, the immediate and late outcomes and consequences of being born small. The NDBC successfully researched into it and established its prevalence, the heterogeneity of LBW with prevalence of both preterm and intrauterine growth-retarded infants (IUGR). It confirmed that a very large proportion of LBW infants are growth retarded and, hence, supported the contention of rationalizing the need of newborns needing care in special care newborn nurseries.

It pointed to the fact that the birthing pattern or the gravidogram differs from the developed countries. The cohort women delivered earlier and most of preterm births occurred as late preterm and at 36 weeks of gestation. The term births occurred at 38–39 weeks rather than at 40 weeks. These observations indicated a strong need for intensive in-depth investigation into the problem of the shift of gravidogram or gestation curve to left resulting in births of large number of preterm and IUGR infants.

The follow-up indicated better survival status due to generally better education, socio-economic status, environment, and sanitation. But the LBW in general and both preterm and SGA suffered in physical growth and CD. These LBW infants over a life course showed significant nutritional handicap and stunting at 5 years of age. They suffered from cardiometabolic disorders in significant numbers. The life course study strongly suggested investing in the policy for prevention of LBW rather than providing for special care newborn nurseries for their immediate care at birth as preferred option in formulation of national policy.

4. **Child Health**

The NDBC results on vital statistics such as child mortality, immunization, growth and development, family planning, and welfare offered insight into the actual happenings and reasons for the dismal prevalent situation of that time. These observations provided hard data towards making some strategies to deal with high mortality rates, poor immunization status, nutrition, failure of family planning programme, creation of growth norms, and assessment of growth failures and child development.

a. **Child survival**

The NDBC childhood mortality rates showed a vast difference between published reports of government and non-government sources. This has been due to the fact that the NDBC data was collected through a trained and committed research team. The NDBC recorded perinatal and neonatal infant and under-five mortality rates, which were high and unacceptable even for that period.

The perinatal and neonatal mortality rates were high due to large proportion of deliveries being conducted at home by untrained or semi-trained health professionals. The high institutional mortality was due to poor efforts in sensitizing women to attend antenatal clinics and poor delivery rooms and neonatal care facilities. It pointed to absence of basic newborn care needs in delivery rooms, neonatal care units, and nurseries and referral to secondary and tertiary level nurseries at an institutional level.

The infant and young child deaths were due to infections such as diarrhoea, respiratory infections, and fevers. The underlying causes were poor environmental conditions and living conditions with overcrowding, poor sanitation, and non-availability of portable and drinking water. The poor socio-economic status and educational levels contributed to it. These observations lent support to the view that reduction in child mortality has to be dealt at multiple levels with equal priority to environment, sanitation, maternal education, and healthcare facilities. The social factors contributing to these had to be dealt by social interventions including educating public and sensitizing them. The NDBC observations lent support to the development of an under-five child health programme which was at that time not discussed as its implications for child health were not understood.

b. **Breastfeeding**

Breastfeeding was universally accepted by the NDBC mothers, but the tendency to introduce artificial milk or top milk seemed to be inherent. There seemed to be a belief that it is the bottle milk which fattens the baby or makes them look chubby. Literacy did not seem to influence the breastfeeding practices. The artificial or top feeding methods and understanding was very frequently wrong. Supplementation with buffalo/cow/powdered milk was early. The milk was often diluted to 50% and introduction of complementary semi-solid/solid food was delayed.

This pointed to the poor and inadequate knowledge about infant feeding. A massive community health education programme directed to sensitize the mother to initiate and sustain breastfeeding till 6 months of infant age and introduce complementary semi-solid feeds after 6 months with locally available or homemade food was required. The unhealthy and mistaken infant feeding practices which are the root causes of malnutrition in children required to be dealt as a major public health programme.

c. **Childhood immunization**

Immunization rates were appallingly low. These were more so in poor income groups and in children born to mothers with poor education and home delivery. The results suggested the need for awareness and sensitization of the population to the benefits of immunization programme and the availability of vaccines.

The continued low and incomplete immunization rates even in present time indicate the need for greater public awareness, availability and strengthening of school health programme from prenursery onwards, and a regulation for compliance of recommended vaccinations by the government in school health programmes. Social interventions will include emphasis on female literacy and promote positive aspects of vaccinations. The myth that it is dangerous and may cause disease or restrict family has to be dealt by appropriate public health education.

5. **Cognitive Development**

Cognitive developmental assessment scales suitable for testing Indian children were not available, we had to modify, adapt, or develop the developmental scales. Several factors influenced the child development at 4 years of age, the most important being maternal education, exposure in preschool nursery. and socio-economic status of family. The results of this study suggested development of appropriate CD scale suitable for Indian children. It also recommended that there is strong evidence to suggest that preschool nursery education improved cognition and suggested provision of preschool nursery facilities for all children from 3 years of age.

6. **Nutrition**

The studies of the NDBC revealed the serious problem of malnutrition. The under-five children were underweight, wasted, or stunted (short in height). All three forms were seen from birth to 5 years. Wasting seemed to decrease after birth and underweight after 2 years, but stunting increased with age. Stunting is known to influence human development with immediate and long-term consequences.

The NDBC studies established foetal to under-five malnutrition as serious childhood problems and recommended foetal growth monitoring by ultrasonography and child growth monitoring from birth to 5 years for an early diagnosis of growth failure.

7. **Age-independent Measurement of Undernutrition**

The NDBC explored in detail the age-independent indices as it was not uncommon to be in situations in the country where simple measurement tools for weight were not available or reliable. The NDBC provided norms for diagnosis of undernutrition in community by measuring mid upper-arm circumference by a tape measure and offered cut off points for its diagnosis.

8. **Growth**

The NDBC's most significant and unique contribution has been through its growth studies. It established for the first time growth curves from birth to 20 years for an urban, Indian community by a prospective well-designed study when measurements were obtained at specific age by trained anthropologists. The curves were developed for linear physical growth, incremental growth, and growth velocity for weight, height, head circumference, and sitting height. The construction of curves offered an opportunity to calculate the BMI. The longitudinal nature of the study allowed growth curves to be broken into different age periods of childhood and to study their effect in adult life. This kind of data was not available in Indian literature and only few studies in world literature made this study unique.

The application of growth curves is not only useful for monitoring of the growth but also for comparison with other similar studies. These studies made it possible to follow through adult life and investigate its association with adult diseases and human capital development. The body weight, height, and BMI observations in relation to size at birth, birth weight, and growth at different periods of childhood adolescence and adulthood made it possible to investigate Barker's hypothesis and developmental origin of adult disease in the NDBC.

# 3

# Childhood Growth, Adult Health, and Human Capital

1. **Childhood Growth, Body Composition, and Adult Diseases**
   Body growth from birth weight to 20 years of age has been related to its association with chronic adult diseases such as diabetes, heart diseases, blood pressure, and metabolic syndrome. The studies demonstrated that those Indian children who were born small (LBW) were thin as young child, got overweight or obese later, and became prone to develop diabetes, hypertension, triglyceride imbalance, and metabolic syndrome as young adults. It was possible to track these diseases on BMI growth curves from as early an age as 2 years onwards by tracking their BMI. The children would become susceptible or develop disease after they begin to cross their path of growth centiles. It was shown for hypertension from early childhood and from mid-childhood and adolescence for dyslipidaemia, glucose imbalance, diabetes, and metabolic syndrome. Overweight and obesity can be tracked from BMI growth charts from early childhood.

   In another study, it was demonstrated that birth weight had an inverse relationship with adult glucose concentrations, impaired fasting glucose, and diabetes mellitus. It has also been pointed out that high birth weight may also be a precursor or may be associated with type II diabetes.

   The results clearly show that it is possible to track these disorders from birth weight and growth charts of the population or use a standard chart like the WHO MGRSs from an early age and get alarmed from the time the child crosses his 50th centile and/or at the beginning of the onset of overweight. The results also emphasized clearly the need to monitor LBW children and weight of children from 4 years onward more closely for excessive or rapid weight gain. Such children can be kept under close supervision and advised appropriate interventions at the earliest.

Body composition was related to birth weight, gestational age, IUGR, BMI, and BMI gain from early childhood to adulthood, and it was recorded that birth weight was directly related to lean mass. In women, a higher birth weight was related to adiposity (fat mass).

Distinct patterns were seen with BMI gain throughout the entire period of childhood growth. Gain in BMI in early infancy and childhood resulted in a gain in lean mass, and a gain in BMI throughout the childhood was associated with adult adiposity and central obesity.

The NDBC studies established association of cardiac risk pro-inflammatory and prothrombotic cardiovascular disease markers with birth weight and BMI gains from 2 years age to adulthood with cardiovascular diseases. It was found that an adverse relationship existed between these markers and the centile crossing of the growth trajectory.

All these observations point to the need of closely monitoring the body growth on standard reference charts. Any aberration or deviation upwards from its own centile growth trajectory should be regarded as a signal for close monitoring of cardiovascular diseases, metabolic syndrome, glucose imbalance, or diabetes.

The NDBC recorded rapid increase in the incidence of obesity, diabetes, hypertension, and IGT within two time periods ranging between 4 and 7 years. There was a significant increase in all of these. The results document an alarming rapid increase in these adult disorders pointing to the need of surveillance and appropriate interventions to prevent the disease or its worsening. It confirms the worst fears that India is on verge of a metabolic and cardiovascular disease epidemic, which will require enormous resources to tackle.

The NDBC also investigated risk factors for conditions predisposing to occurrence of CAD and stroke. This involved ultrasound studies of the vessel walls of carotid artery located in the neck, which showed significant presence of plaques. A positive association was found between CIMT and increased waist measurement, longer body length, high diastolic blood pressure, triglycerides, PAI-1, insulin resistance, metabolic syndrome, and lower HDL.

The data supported the relevance of a simple measure such as waist circumference measurement and preventive cardiac checkup for early diagnosis of factors predisposing to causation of heart disease and stroke.

2. **Growth Monitoring, Health, and Disease**

From the NDBC studies, it strongly follows that growth monitoring, and not just recording, should be made mandatory. If properly monitored and interpreted, it may help in counselling the parents at appropriate time for intervention.

Foetal and childhood period growth monitoring appears to be key to future health. Foetal growth monitoring is poor across the country. The nation may consider adopting INTERGROWTH-21 as a reference for foetal growth and follow the foetal growth on these intrauterine growth curves. These are developed by WHO through an international multi-country study of which India was also a part. These may be considered as a reference but not as a standard.

From birth, the children should be monitored for their growth on the IAP growth reference charts, or Government of India growth curves, or the WHO growth curves which are now well accepted.

The national child nutrition policy also needs to be implemented with different focus and attention. It should be vigorously pursued to attain maximal positive body size gain in first 2 years by nutrition support, if necessary, and health measures. Thereafter, the emphasis in the childhood and schooling period should be to maintain normal growth and to intensify growth monitoring to detect centile crossing.

In the national Integrated Child Development Services (ICDS) programme, the emphasis and focus should be more on first two years as it has positive gains for childhood and adulthood health and human capital development. The mid-day meal focus should be to ensure correction of growth deficit through adequate nutrition.

Growth monitoring can be effectively done through the school health programme. As per Central Board of Secondary Education (CBSE) directive, every child has to have an annual health examination by the school health service. These are done, but unfortunately the growth data is not interpreted properly or interpreted inadequately or even incorrectly. The NDBC data suggest the urgent need to do effective growth monitoring in ICDS programme which uses a health card, and schools which also use health cards. National growth charts by IAP, Government of India, Ministry of Health and Welfare, and WHO are available. These should be uniformly used and incorporated in health records. Growth monitoring along with recording of blood pressure and other measures should be compulsory for all schools and the records with interpretation by school health professional reported to parents.

3. **Childhood Growth and Human Capital Development**

The NDBC growth data strongly correlated with human capital development. Adult height showed a strong association with length at birth and conditional length at 24 months of age. It was strongly affected by growth failure in the first year. Adult stature was related to income generation.

The NDBC studies showed that birth weight, weight gain in 0–24 months and 24–48 months, and stunting significantly influenced the schooling outcome. It showed weight gain in 0–24 months increases schooling which increased the income by 10%. An increase in birth weight showed an increase in schooling years, decreased chances of failure in a grade or class, and increased chances of completing schooling. Thus weight gain in the first 2 years offers tremendous benefits for later life.

In a pooled analysis of the COHORTS group, birth weight, faster gain in height, a faster relative weight, linear growth, and relative weight gain influenced adult health and well-being. Higher birth weight was associated with higher BMI and decreased risk of short adult stature and decreased chances of completing school education. Faster gain in height decreased the chances of short adult stature but increased the risk of overweight and high blood pressure. A faster weight gain was associated with higher risk of overweight and blood pressure. Higher birth weight decreased the risk of glucose imbalance.

These observations clearly demonstrate the usefulness of birth weight, weight, height, and BMI growth trajectory to identify possible risk of adult disease and human capital. It emphasizes the need to monitor growth from birth to adulthood and its implications.

4. **Influence of Maternal and Child Undernutrition and Human Capital Development**

In a pioneering study, the COHORTS group studied the influence of maternal size, birth weight, foetal growth restriction, and BMI at 2 years of age and related these to adult outcomes of final attained height, schooling, income generation, and birth weight of next generation. It showed that growth restriction in intrauterine life and first 2 years adversely affected the adult outcome.

Height significantly influences the schooling outcome. Birth weight of offspring of the mother is influenced by growth between 0 and 24 months but is not affected by later growth. The study demonstrated the adverse influence of growth failure in first 2 years and the importance of monitoring it in this period, which appears to be most critical for human development.

The observations on foetal intrauterine growth and the first 2 years of life perhaps led to the coining of the term 'first 1,000 days' as this period seems to influence the outcome from birth to adulthood and later life.

# 4

# Intergeneration and Trans-generational Changes

1. **Intergeneration**

   The intergeneration studies on influence of socio-economic, education, cultural, and environmental changes have shown striking changes, which influenced several outcome measures of the NDBC and their children of next generations. It recorded positive socio-cultural change, income generation, environment and sanitation improvement, educational and occupation change, and lifestyle changes in both male and female cohorts. The change improved certain health parameters but also showed a possible deterioration for adult diseases due to lifestyle changes. Thus, all socio-economic, educational, and environmental factors should be periodically reviewed to explain changes or emergence of disease pattern.

   One of the most important trans-generation changes was seen in the anthropometric measurement of weight, height, and BMI between cohorts who are parents and F1 generation and of their children or F2 generation at the same age. A positive change was seen at all age periods of childhood in weight, height, and BMI. The positive change indicates the need of intergeneration studies and detailed explorations as to what effected the change in a negative or positive way.

   The F2 generation had marginally low mean birth weight compared to their parents. However, the LBW prevalence declined from 20.8% to 18.0% in the F2 generation. The decline in prevalence of LBW infants in the same family, living in the same albeit better environment, indicate a trans-generational change and questions the need to interfere with the natural course.

Both undernutrition and overnutrition recorded significant intergenerational changes between the F1 and F2 generations. Undernutrition in the first five years recorded a sharp decline of wasting in first two years but an increase in the fourth and fifth years. Stunting declined throughout the five years but was striking in the first two years. Underweight continued to decline throughout the first five years.

The increase in wasting in the fourth and fifth years pointed to the need of further detailed study. The change across the first five years in undernutrition in two generations again points to importance of intergenerational studies while planning strategies to improve the situation.

An increase in prevalence of overweight throughout the childhood in F2 was of concern and needs to be studied in detail. However, this generation is going through a change in lifestyle, family wealth, and nutritional habits and nutrition availability.

2. **Trans-generation**

The trans-generation study on sleep disorders and its association with cardiometabolic risk factors demonstrated an increasing deteriorating scene with generational change from F0 to F1 and to F2 of the three generations of the NDBC. Risk factors such as overweight, obesity, glucose intolerance, hypertension, and lipid aberrations developed earlier and their prevalence increased with advancing age in the three generations. These seemed to be related to nutritional and lifestyle transition and suggested the need to initiate tracking of these diseases from early age through the monitoring of cardiometabolic risk factors by appropriate clinical and laboratory tests.

3. **Third Generation Children**

In the third generation or children of the NDBC cohort, specific disorders were investigated. Occurrence of overweight, obesity, hypertension, IGT, and lipid aberrations showed the children to be affected in significant numbers and from a younger age. Behavioural disorders were seen in almost every other child. The severity of behaviour changes affected the scholastic performance of the children. Mother's education, spending time on computer, and TV viewing predisposed to this occurrence. The results suggested the adverse influence of the lifestyle changes and indicated the need to investigate these disorders with alacrity on aberration in growth pattern and deteriorating or poor school grades and performance.

# 5

# Challenges to Community Participation

1. **Attrition and the Loss to Follow-Up**
   The NDBC had suffered significant loss of cohort. Almost 75% of the cohorts were lost in the long follow-up. This is not unexpected in a study of this kind which is community-based in a metropolitan city, and it is consistent with the experience of similar cohorts.
   One of the main reasons was interruptions due to discontinuation of research grants and the inordinate time it took to get the sanction for the continuation of the research. The shifting of the research office several times and lack of a permanent office also contributed to attrition. The cohort fatigue and marked improvement in availability in private sector were some of the other reasons.

2. **Community Participation and Expectations**
   The community participation could have been enhanced in the project by better understanding of their needs and more personal interaction between participants, the research team, and investigators. The medical issues which the cohorts had could not be addressed due to nature of the study. It was agreed in the beginning that no intervention or medical advice will be offered. This was a major constrain. Finally, the project objectives, necessity, advantages, and drawbacks must be explained repeatedly. This will increase the perceptions of the participants which will go a long way in building mutual trust.

# PART 9

# **Summation**

# Introduction

The New Delhi Birth Cohort was established in 1969 as a collaborative research project 'Outcome and Survival of a Birth Cohort' by a grant from PL 480 funds to Dr Shanti Ghosh and Dr Santosh K. Bhargava from Safdarjung Hospital, New Delhi, India, and Dr I. M. Moriyama from the National Centre for Health and Statistics, USA. It was founded to investigate the problem of LBW in India in a comprehensive manner including prevalence, survival, and sequelae amongst the surviving children.

It was a difficult time for conducting research in India as appropriate resources in terms of equipment, trained manpower; data storage, and analysis were not available. The project had to develop and fabricate the equipment such as weighing and height measuring scales locally, train the staff, and use manually operated tools and manpower to store the data. It used a repaired calculating machine for routine work and data analysis. Later on, computers became available and the same were used. The entire study was protocol based and standard operating procedures were used.

A well-defined 12 sq km area in South Delhi—Lajpat Nagar—was selected for the project. The population of the selected area was 119,799 with 20,755 ever-married women in the reproductive age between 13 and 49 years. These women were followed up every 2 months + 3 days to ascertain the LMP, and any woman missing the period was followed as a possible pregnancy. Thus, ever-married, non-pregnant women were followed from pregnancy to the birth of the cohort. The infants thus born constituted the NDBC.

## Profile of Ever-married Women

There were 20,755 ever-married women, but only those between 13 and 49 years of age and reproductively active were followed. In case of a missed period, pregnancy was confirmed and the woman was followed as per pregnancy protocol. About 43% of the women were less than 19 years. Most of them were from the middle-income group and were literates. The fertility pattern revealed interesting findings. Majority were married by 18 years of age and had a fertility period of 20 years or more. Around 25% of them had five or more pregnancies and the mean number of pregnancies was 3.56. Teenage marriage was common and seen in all religions. Education and income influenced the age at marriage directly in a positive way.

Cohabitation occurred within one year of marriage and was more common in educated women. The first child was usually born within 2 years of marriage. The age at marriage, per capita income, and religion did not influence the number of pregnancies. Interestingly, the number of pregnancies increased with the number of foetal death or child deaths. The mean interval between two consecutive pregnancies was 2.6 years.

Family planning practices showed that 29.9% were using contraceptive method and an overwhelming 70.1% were not using any family planning method. Contraceptives were the method of choice till 35 years of age and sterilization was used more commonly thereafter. Education and income were directly related to family planning practices. The most significant finding was the influence of foetal death or child mortality. Even with one death, the family planning practice showed a decline, and after 3 or more deaths the family planning practice was discontinued.

## Pregnancy

Pregnancies were recorded in 9,509 women. Antenatal registration was done by 75% of women. But the antenatal visits in general were unsatisfactory. Stillbirths were seen in 2.09%. Majority of the women delivered at their predetermined place of choice. Institution or facility-based deliveries were recorded in 60%, and 40% births occurred at home.

## The Birth of the Cohorts

A total of 8,181 cohorts were born at different places of births. Amongst these, 8,030 were single births, 74 twins, and one triplet. About 71.6% of the infants were born term, 16.4% preterm, and 12.4% as term infants. The mean birth weight was 2,790 g.

# Low Birth Weight

The LBW (<2,500 g) prevalence was high at 26.2%, with 22.2% weighing between 2,001 and 2,499 g. Important predictors of LBW included poor environment and sanitation, maternal pregravid weight and height, poor nutrition, teenage pregnancy, birth interval of less than 2 years, poor education, and income.

Amongst the LBW, 81.2% were AGA, 9.4% were SGA, and 9.2% were LGA. Stunting was seen in 8.9%. The mortality was high and inversely related to birth weight and gestational age—the lower the birth weight and gestational age the higher the mortality

Birth weight and gestation influenced future physical growth and CD. They remained small throughout the childhood period. The CD was also affected and in adulthood; both preterm and LBW SGA had less schooling as compared to normal term AGA children.

Over 300 LBW children could be followed from birth to 45 years of age. Amongst these children, maternal education did not influence the birth weight. The mothers were employed in a variety of professions from homemakers to skilled jobs, managers, service, and professional workers and were comparable to mothers of normal weight children. Undernutrition was seen to be common in all three forms of wasting, underweight, and stunting. Stunting was a major problem at 2–3 years which continued till 5 years of age. Cardiometabolic disorders were seen as hypertension (26.4%), high cholesterol (56.4%), high triglycerides (44.5%), and diabetes (14.5%). It was comparable to normal weight children. This was a small sample study; a large-population-based study is needed to confirm these findings.

## Child Survival, Health and Disease

The neonatal, infant, and under-five mortality rates as compared to nation and Delhi state for that time were low, but quite high. LBW and preterm seemed to contribute maximally to child mortality, while diarrhoea and respiratory infections were common morbidities. Congenital malformations were seen in 26.2 per 1,000 births and musculo-skeletal malformations were common. CNS malformations were the most common major malformation.

Immunization rates were low and only small pox vaccination was seen in over 95%. Three doses of DPT and Polio were received by 50–60% children. Immunization rates were higher in institution-based deliveries and educated parents.

## Growth

Growth studies were the highlight of the NDBC research. Growth was evaluated from birth to 20 years at an age-specific period with trained anthropologists recording the measurements. The data encompasses all age periods from birth to adulthood with birth weight, first 2 years, mid childhood, adolescence, and adult growth measurements, which included linear physical growth and incremental growth for weight, height, head circumference, and sitting height. Body composition measurements of skinfold thickness from multiple sites and waist circumference were also recorded.

The NDBC has constructed body growth curves for both genders from birth to 20 years for weight, height, and head circumference and also incremental growth charts. The factors influencing growth were birth weight, gestation, income, environment factors, and childhood nutrition.

## Cognitive Development

The CD was studied at three different periods of childhood. It was recorded in infancy and second year and selectively for children with birth weight of 2,000 g or less at 4 and 6 years. The CD was affected in LBW, SGA, and preterm infants. The most significant finding was the distinct influence of preschool or nursery schooling.

## Nutrition

Undernutrition was a very major problem and overnutrition was hardly seen. In undernutrition, all three types, namely, wasting, underweight, and stunting were seen. Severe form of undernutrition was less common. The most affected period in all three norms was birth weight and 2–3 years of age. Stunting was a striking major problem and was seen in 50% by 2 years of age. Severe stunting was seen in 10–20% of the children and was most frequent at 2–3 years. Female children were more affected than male children.

In the NDBC children, MUAC was also recorded as a surrogate measure for identification of undernutrition in community and maternal and child health centres where weighing scales are not available.

## Transition to Adult Phase

The childhood phase was completed in 1991 with most of the cohort attaining an age of 20 years. The project was officially closed as almost all the objectives as defined from time to time in different phases were completed.

In 1994, the writer Professor Bhargava, Professor Barker, and Dr Fall had a meeting and it was decided to revive the project by re-establishing contact with the cohort.

## The Adult Phase

The adult phase was started in 1998–2002 with a grant from the British Heart Foundation. This investigated Barker's hypothesis and the influence of childhood growth on development of adult disease such as diabetes, hypertension, metabolic syndrome, and others. It showed that it is possible to track these diseases by tracking childhood growth and BMI.

Thereafter, several grants were received from national and international funding agencies. The most notable amongst these was our joining with the four other low middle-income countries with similar cohorts to form a consortium of health oriented research in transiting societies (COHORTS). These included Pelotas (Brazil), INCAP (Guatemala), Cebu (Philippines), and BT 20 (South Africa). We investigated the influence of birth weight and body growth in early, middle childhood, and adolescence to adulthood on cardiometabolic disorder, human capital development, final stature, schooling, income generation, and birth weight of the next offspring.

## Changing Socio-Cultural and Environmental Characteristics in the Adult Phase

In 1,583 cohorts, we were able to obtain information on socio-cultural and environmental characteristics and were able to compare the same with their parent's status when they were born (1969–73).

About 75% of the cohorts were married and had nuclear families. Many lived in flats or independents houses. Almost all were educated with over 40% as graduate and professional, and this number had doubled as compared to their parents. Occupation had undergone change with almost all being now skilled workers, in business, self-employed, or class I officers. Only 1/4th or 26.6% of women were housewives as compared to over 75% in 1969–73. Around 20% cohorts were also engaged in secondary business.

The cohorts' wealth status had changed. Almost all had electric fans, radios and televisions, air coolers, electric mixers, and gas stoves and 30–50% now owned scooters, motor cycles, cars, and air conditioners.

The women were no more doing only household chores, fetching water and firewood, or impounding cattle. They went for jogs, morning walks, yoga, exercise, and other leisure activities like watching TV serials.

Inter-caste marriages had become common. Teenage marriage had declined. Many languages were being spoken at home, but Hindi was the dominant language. About 60% of the families were non-vegetarian. Walking was the predominant mode of exercise and a few went to gymnasiums.

## Medical History

It was surprising to find a host of illness in young adults. Hypertension was the most common and others included tuberculosis, diabetes, respiratory problems, and the occasional cerebral stroke. The families took different kinds of treatment from different systems of medical practice. Mental stress and anxiety were emerging problems.

## New Delhi Birth Cohort Research

### Childhood Growth, Adult Health, and Diseases

1. **Size at Birth, Birth Weight, BMI, Growth in Childhood and Adult Diseases**

As mentioned earlier, it is possible to track adult diseases such as IGT, diabetes, hypercholesterolemia, dyslipidaemia, and hypertension by tracking growth on standard growth and BMI charts. Children who are thin at 2 years and have rapid growth, or children with rapid gain in BMI, or those who tend to cross their growth trajectories above their 50th centile are potentially at risk for these diseases.

2. **BMI and Adult Metabolic Syndrome**
   The NDBC investigated the possibility of identifying children at risk of developing adult metabolic syndrome through BMI charts. This was possible, and it recorded a high (29.0%) prevalence of metabolic syndrome.

3. **Size at Birth, BMI Body Composition, and Chronic Adult Diseases**
   Birth weight was directly related to lean mass, suggesting that higher birth weight newborns have higher lean mass. In women, higher birth weight was related to adiposity (fatness) but not to central obesity (waist circumference). Higher BMI and higher BMI gain recorded different patterns. Higher BMI in children was associated with higher adult BMI (obesity) and higher waist-hip ratio (large waist). BMI and BMI gains were associated with adult lean mass. These observations strongly suggested that it is possible to track obesity through BMI tracking from childhood.

   In another similar study, birth weight and weight trajectories through the first 24 months or 2 years were strongly associated with fat-free mass. On the other hand, weight trajectories in mid-childhood predicted both fat mass and lean mass, but the latter more than the former.

   In yet another study on size at birth and body growth, it was found that bone size was strongly related to height and weight at birth and height growth in infancy. The bone density was strongly related to BMI and BMI gain during childhood and adolescence.

4. **Cardiovascular Diseases**
   The childhood body growth and BMI were significantly associated with cardiovascular diseases including hypertension and carotid artery plaques. The study on CVS pro-inflammatory and pro-thrombotic markets showed an association with birth weight and BMI gain after 2 years and adolescence.

   In another study of body growth and body composition with CVS risk factors and cardiometabolic disease in two successive follow-up with a gap of 6–8 years, an association was found with waist circumference, hip circumference, systolic and diastolic pressure, lipids, and cholesterols. In general, women showed higher rate of increase of obesity but the men dominated in diabetes and hypertension in successive follow-ups after 6–8 years of interval. The incidence of diabetes and hypertension almost doubled during this short period, forewarning of impending cardiometabolic disorders epidemic onslaught in our population.

In a study on carotid arteries—large blood vessels supplying blood to brain—their vessel wall showed plaques in over 30%. A positive association of this was found with waist circumference. A longer body length at 2 years was also associated with the vessel wall CIMT. These observations again suggested the usefulness of a simple anthropometric measurement like waist circumference in the tracking of such diseases.

5. **Body Growth and Human Capital Development**
   Human capital development was assessed by attainment of adult stature, schooling and its grades, income generation, and the birth weight in the next generation offspring in pooled analyses of COHORTS group. The birth weight and length, body growth from 0–24 months and 24–48 months, and length at 2 years were related to final adult stature and schooling.

   It showed that birth weight, weight gain in 0–24 months and 24–48 months, and the occurrence of stunting significantly influenced the schooling outcome such as enrolment age in school, failure in any grades during schooling, and completing schooling. An increase in weight gain by 1 SD between 0 and 24 months was associated with an increase in income generation by 10%. An increase in birth weight showed an increase in schooling years and decrease in chances of failure in school grade.

   The influence of birth weight, weight gain and linear growth at different periods of childhood was related to metabolic syndrome, diabetes, and cardiometabolic disorders. The cohort group also found that higher birth weight was associated with higher BMI and decreased risk of short stature and not completing secondary school. Faster gain in height decreased the chances of short adult stature and chances of not completing schooling education. But this increased the risk of overweight and elevated blood pressure.

   The influence of maternal size, birth weight, foetal growth, and the individual weight, height, and BMI at 2 years of age was related to adult outcome of final attained height, schooling, income generation, and birth weight of next generation offspring by the cohort group. Growth failure in the intrauterine period and first two years significantly influenced the adult height, but not thereafter. Birth weight and weight gain in 0–24 months had the strongest influence on schooling higher grade attainment, grade failure, and age at school entry. Weight gain during 0–12 months had the strongest influence followed by birth weight. Weight gain during 24–48 months had the least influence on schooling outcome.

The foetal growth period and the first 24 months' life are considered the most critical period of human life and this led to the coining of the term 'the first 1,000 days.'

## Intergeneration and Trans-generation

The NDBC is now a four-generation family cohort. The F0 are parents of cohorts, F1 the cohorts, F2 the children of cohorts, and F3 the grandchildren of cohorts.

In the F0 generation, more fathers have died than mothers, suggesting longer life for women. In F1 generation, the sex ratio is the same; but in F2 generation, greater number of male children is seen as compared to female children. This is a distinct change as compared to the previous generation and shows a preference for male children.

In anthropometry, a striking change is seen in favour of the children of cohorts or F2 generation. It shows a gain in F2 favour with an increase in body measurements. A clear change was seen in SD scores of weight, height, and BMI. The change in weight was from 0.8 to 1.3 SD, in height the change was from 0.7 to 1.2 SD, and in BMI from 0.3 to 1.1 SD. The change was observed between 5 and 12.5 years of age.

The prevalence of LBW also showed a significant decrease from 20.8% in F1 to 18% (p < 001) in F2 generation.

The most significant intergenerational change was seen in the malnutrition profile of F1 and F2 generations. While undernutrition in all the three forms decreased, overnutrition was seen as overweight and obesity in all age groups of F2 generation. The maximum decline in wasting occurred at birth and in first 2 years. The stunting decreased throughout the five-year period but was sharp in the first 2 years. The underweight also declined sharply in second year.

The BMI had shown a change throughout the childhood period, suggesting an increase in occurrence of overweight and obesity in children as this was hardly seen in F1 generation.

The trans-generation changes appear to be related to improvement in environment, sanitation, education, nutrition, and positive health measures like immunization in childhood.

Trans-generation disorder in the three generations F0, F1, and F2 was selectively studied for sleep disorders. Grandparents slept the least number of hours with grandmothers sleeping the least and the children the most. All adult diseases such as hypertension, obesity, and dyslipidaemia increased with age. Snoring was the most common sleep-associated disorder.

## The Third Generation

Three thousand seven hundred and fifty two children were tracked in the third or F2 generation of the NDBC. About 1,000 children were investigated for selective cardiovascular, sleep, and behaviour disorders. The mean birth weight was 2,817.2 g and LBW prevalence was 18%. menarche occurred between 10 and 13 years but was mostly seen to occur at 13 and 14 years of age.

The cardiovascular risk factor study showed prevalence of overweight in 25% with 5.3% as obese. Central obesity or increased waist size was seen in 22.4%, and prehypertension varied from 10–18% in boys and girls. Hypertension was seen in 7.7% but was three time more common in girls. IGT and hyper-triglyceridemia was seen in 10% and low HDL prevalence in 23.5%. It was alarming to see this high prevalence of cardiovascular risk factors in adolescent children.

Sleep disorder was studied in two groups of 4–12 and 12–18 years. The children went off to sleep easily. The bed time and waking time was delayed on weekends. TV watching increased over weekends. Parasomnia was the common group of symptoms with grinding of teeth, nightmares, enuresis, and sleep walking in 4–12 age group children and snoring was common.

Behaviour problem were studied in 200 F2 children using CBCL and CGAS. Behaviour problems were very common and were seen in 48% of children. Low maternal education, long TV-watching hours, and time spent on computer was associated with behavioural problems. A spectrum of disorders was seen varying from depression, enuresis, anxiety, and aggressive, defiant, and diligent behaviour.

Handgrip strength study was done to determine its relationship with birth weight and adult health. Two ninety children of 10–19 years were investigated. A significant association was found between grip strength and anthropometry, body composition (BMI, fat mass, and lean mass), and systolic and diastolic blood pressures. However, there was no significant association with metabolic variables such as fasting blood glucose, cholesterol, HDL, LDL, and triglycerides.

## Attrition or Loss to Follow-up

Attrition in this study was expected to be high and significant. The cohort were 8,181 in numbers to begin with in 1969. We have currently traced 2,148 cohort, in the last round of census in 2015. There is thus a loss of over 6,037 (73.7%) of the cohort. This is high because of several reasons but is mainly due to demolition of a number of housing colonies in the 1970s with loss of over 2,000 cohorts. The other reasons are deaths, migrations, and interruptions in follow-up due to lack of research funding. An important underlying reason is the community behaviour. The cohort did not leave a forwarding address nor informed us, nor did they post the self-addressed stamped letters. The cohorts were cooperative, but due to design of the study we could not offer any medical assistance or intervention. We also did not compensate the cohort for their time or travel.

Social factors like not letting the in-laws know about their long follow-up caused fear in the minds of women and their parents. The cohorts got married and shifted their homes within the city, in India, or abroad. The frequent change of staff, the weather, and school vacations also contributed to attrition. A very possible factor could be cohort fatigue due to repeated visits and the same set of questions and enquiries.

## Cohorts Participation, Expectations, and Challenges

We were indeed extremely fortunate to get this kind of cooperation and participation by the members of the NDBC. It is surprising that despite an entirely voluntary participation with no compensation in cash or kind, we received an overwhelming and wholehearted support from those cohorts whom we could reach. We did not have to use much persuasion or spend time in convincing. They were for some reason committed to participate in the studies. Many believed it to be their duty. They had implicit trust and faith in us. They felt very strongly that we will do no harm and that this was not for monetary benefits for the research team. They strongly felt that whatever we will do it will be good for them, for the community, and for medical science. A strong bond of trust between the cohorts and us was key to the success of their cooperation and participation.

The initial home-based data collection in the childhood phase and later organization of clinics in the near vicinity and neighbourhood of their homes helped in enhancing participation.

We sent original reports, albeit sometimes late, but always ensured that they were received by them. We interpreted the reports for them and always advised them to consult their physician. We organized interactive meetings with investigators so that they could meet and know them personally and we maintained absolute confidentiality. A strong reason could also be the association of staff who served the project for many years and some of them for more than 30 years.

In spite of all these, some subjects refused to participate for a number of reasons. These included indifference, mistakenly taking us for other health workers, long waiting hours in clinic for tests, environment of clinic, late reports, communication failure, ethical issues, misinformation, faiths, and beliefs. At times, the sheer fear of blood collection made them refuse or run away from the clinic.

## Implication and Impact

The NDBC research project is one of the oldest cohorts from a low middle-income country with women followed prospectively from pre-pregnant state to pregnancy to childbirth, childhood, and adulthood, and it is presently in its fifth decade of a continuous follow-up. It was unique for its time and path breaking in many ways. It developed and fabricated its own research tools, protocols, training methods and quality standards, and data depository. We collected and analysed data manually, then by calculators, and were one of the first users of early generation computers. It is a dynamic project, which adapted and modified its objectives and methodology with time to remain relevant to community and country needs.

When the NDBC was established, cohort research was not in vogue nor was it attempted. However, it is currently the flavour of global research.

We focused on public health problems. These were LBW, fertility, and family planning, and childhood mortality. The cohort had high fertility rates caused by illiteracy, child and teenage marriage, and large families due to high child mortality. Cohabitation occurred within a year of marriage and the first child was born in first 2 years. The mean interval between two pregnancies was more than 2 years. Child mortality affected the family planning. Its practice declined with foetal or child death and couples abandoned the family planning totally with three deaths or more. Education and income directly influenced family planning practices.

These findings clearly sent the message of improving maternal education, focusing on social interventions to avoid child and teenage marriage and first pregnancy, and increasing time interval between two successive pregnancies. The striking influence of child mortality experience pointed to an urgent need to improve child survival status and ensure child survival. Child survival became a national programme in the 1980s and 1990s. The government also adopted an integrated programme on maternal and child health to control the fertility and to increase family planning acceptance and improve child survival.

The pregnancy registration was high. But antenatal attendance, and therefore antenatal care, was poor. More than 40% of births occurred at home by trained, semi-trained, or untrained health professionals.

Newborns died in large numbers and were the largest contributors to child mortality. This was due to almost non-existent newborn care from primary to higher levels. The immunization rates were low and children suffered from diarrhoea, respiratory infections, and fevers.

The issue of LBW was studied extensively and comprehensively from foetal growth to prevalence, causes, survival, growth, and development. A unique feature was the follow-up of over 300 LBW from birth to 45 years of age.

The data has recorded a high prevalence of LBW with about 16% as preterm and over 85% as intrauterine growth retarded. More than 30% of preterm births occur at 36 weeks and more births occur at 37, 38, and 39 weeks, and over 85% of LBW is between 2,001 and 2,499 g. The foetal growth begins to flatten from 34 weeks. These findings strongly suggest the need to investigate why the onset of labour is earlier in our women and why foetal growth slows from 34 weeks gestation.

The preterm and intrauterine growth-retarded SGA remains small throughout childhood to adulthood. Their CD scores are lower and their final attainment of education is lower than normal term infants.

Almost 40% of low birth children showed occurrence of chronic adult diseases of hypertension, hypercholesterolaemia, dyslipidaemia, and

IGT. All these findings indicate the urgent need to prevent LBW occurrence as it is too expensive to look after them once they are born.

Growth tracking was a unique feature of the NDBC research, with longitudinal recordings from birth to 20 years at age-specific periods by trained anthropologists. It had linear physical growth of weight, height, and head circumference from infancy, early and mid-childhood, adolescence, and adulthood.

The NDBC constructed growth charts, which can be compared to current reference standard of the Indian Academy of Paediatrics or the WHO growth charts. Birth weight, gestation, and income influenced the growth amongst the children.

Development was assessed selectively at 4 and 6 years of age in the same children of LBW. The results suggested a strong case for provision of preschool education for every child.

Nutrition assessment showed malnutrition to be prevalent, with undernutrition being much more common than overnutrition. Undernutrition was seen in all three forms of wasting, underweight, and stunting; these occurred most frequently at 2–3 years of age. Stunting was a much more serious problem and seemed to increase with age.

## The Intergeneration and Trans-generation Studies

The results of the intergeneration and trans-generation studies of birth weight, nutrition, and anthropometric studies showed the increasing need of such studies. These are most helpful to planners and administrators for developing intervention strategies.

The F2 or second generation studies are an eye opener as these indicate the development of cardiometabolic risk factors from 10 to 19 years. Behaviour disorders were seen in almost every other child with a problem suggesting need of parenting and review of schooling methods. The sleep disorders suggest the need for child discipline on sleeping time, sleeping hours, TV viewing, monitoring, and computer time.

The NDBC story has been expanding from its inception. It has moved from a single generation to a four-generation cohort. It has been a dynamic project adapting itself to the changing time. The future seems to be exciting with new collaborations, ever-changing better tools for investigations, analysis, and new investigators joining the NDBC Research Group.

# Appendix

## Suggested Readings: Peer-reviewed Publications from the New Delhi Birth Cohort

### Publications 1969–90

1. Hooja V, Madhavan S, Ahmad SH, Ghosh S. Outcome and survival of a birth cohort in a community of South Delhi: Preliminary report of a prospective study. Indian Pediatr. 1972; 9: 495–505.
2. Ahmad SH, Bhargava SK, Ramanujacharyulu C, Hooja V, Ghosh S, Moriyama IM. Maternal health, child health and family planning: A plea for integrated approach. Indian Pediatr. 1973; 10(11): 637–45.
3. Ghosh S, Hooja V, Ahmad SH, Acharyulu RC, Bhargava SK. A longitudinal study of length, weight and head circumference from birth to 2 years among children of high socio-economic urban community in Delhi. Indian Pediatr. 1974; 11(6): 395–98.
4. Hooja V, Ghosh S, Mittal SK, Verma RK. Immunization status in an urban community. Indian Pediatr. 1976; 13(10): 747–50.
5. Ghosh S, Gidwani S, Mittal SK, Verma RK. Socio-cultural factors affecting breast feeding practices in an urban community. Indian Pediatr. 1976; 13(11): 827–32.
6. Ghosh S, Hooja V, Mittal SK, Verma RK. Bio-social determinants of birth weight. Indian Pediatr. 1977; 14(2): 107–14.
7. Ghosh S, Ramanujacharyulu TK, Hooja V, Madhavan S. Mortality pattern in an urban birth cohort. Indian J Med Res. 1979; 69: 616–23.
8. Bhargava SK, Ghosh S, Lall UB. A study of low birth weight infants in an urban community. Health Popul Perspect Issues. 1979; 2(1): 54–66.
9. Ghosh S, Zaidi I, Lakshmy A, Choudhury P, Bhargava SK. Growth and development of children in different ecological settings. Indian J Nutr Diet. 1979; 16: 155–64.

10. Bhargava SK, Bhargava U, Kumari S, Bhargava N, Ghosh S. Maternal nutrition and fetal growth retardation. J Trop Pediatr. 1983; 29(3): 148–50.

11. Bhargava SK, Kumari S, Choudhury P. Outcome of low birth weight infants. Acta Pediatr Scand. 1984; 73(3): 406–07.

12. Ghosh S, Bhargava SK, Butani R. Congenital malformations in a longitudinally studied birth cohort in an urban community. Indian J Med Res. 1985; 82: 427–33.

13. Bhargava SK, Sachdev HP, Ghosh S. Early neonatal mortality in an urban birth cohort: Relationship to birth weight and gestational age. Indian J Com Med. 1985; 10(1): 11–13.

14. Bhargava SK, Sachdev HP, Ghosh S. Distribution of live births and early neonatal mortality in relation to gestation and intrauterine growth. Indian J Med Res. 1985; 82: 95–97.

15. Bhargava SK, Sachdev HP, Iyer PU, Ramji S. Current status of infant growth measurements in the perinatal period in India. Acta Paediatr Scand Suppl. 1985; 319: 103–10.

16. Bhargava SK, Ramji S, Arun Kumar, Mohan M, Marwah J, Sachdev HP. Mid-arm and chest circumference at birth as predictors of low birth weight and neonatal mortality in the community. Br Med J. 1985; 291(6509): 1617–19.

17. Shrivastava U, Sachdev HP, Bhargava SK, Ghosh S. Morbidity pattern of adolescents in an urban community. Indian Pediatr. 1985; 22(10): 753–56.

18. Bhargava SK, Sachdev HP, Ramji S, Iyer PU. Low birthweight: Aetiology and prevention in India. Ann Trop Paediatr. 1987; 7(1): 59–65.

19. Ghosh S. Infant and childhood mortality. Indian Pediatr. 1987; 24(8): 613–18.

20. Bhargava SK, Sachdev HS, Fall CHD, Osmond C, Lakshmy R, Barker DJP, Biswas SKD, Ramji S, Prabhakaran D, Reddy KS. Relation of serial changes in childhood bodymass index to impaired glucose tolerance in young adulthood. N Engl J Med. 2004; 350: 865–75.

21. Sachdev HS, Fall CHD, Osmond C. The changing face and implications of childhood obesity. N Engl J Med 2004; 350: 2414–16.

22. Sachdev HS, Fall CHD, Osmond C, Lakshmy R, Dey Biswas SK, Leary SD, Reddy KS, Barker DJP, Bhargava SK. Anthropometric indicators of body composition in young adults: Relation to size at birth and serial measurements of body mass index in childhood in the New Delhi birth cohort. Am J Clin Nutr. 2005; 82(2): 456–66.

23. Fall CHD, Sachdev HS, Osmond C, Lakshmy R, Dey Biswas SK, Prabhakaran D, Tandon N, Ramji S, Reddy KS, Barker DJ, Bhargava SK. Adult metabolic syndrome and impaired glucose tolerance are associated with different patterns of body mass index gain during infancy; Data from the New Delhi birth cohort. Diabetes Care. 2008; 31(12): 2349–56.

24. Sachdev HS, Osmond C, Fall CH, Lakshmy R, Ramji S, Dey Biswas S, Prabhakaran D, Tandon N, Reddy KS, Barker DJP, Bhargava SK. Predicting adult metabolic syndrome from childhood body mass index: Follow-up of the New Delhi birth. Arch Dis Child. 2009; 94(10): 768–74.

25. Whincup PH, Kaye SJ, Owen CG, Huxley R, Cook DG, Anazawa S, Barrett-Connor E, Bhargava SK, Birgisdottir BE, Carlsson S, de Rooij SR, Dyck RF, Eriksson JG, Falkner B, Fall C, Forsén T, Grill V, Gudnason V, Hulman S, Hyppönen E, Jeffreys M, Lawlor DA, Leon DA, Minami J, Mishra G, Osmond C, Power C, Rich-Edwards JW, Roseboom TJ, Sachdev HS, Syddall H, Thorsdottir I, Vanhala M,Wadsworth M, Yarbrough DE. Birth weight and risk of type 2 diabetes: A systematic review. JAMA. 2008; 300(24): 2886–97.

26. Victora CG, Adair L, Fall C, Hallal PC, Martorell R, Richter L, Sachdev HS; Maternal and Child Undernutrition Study Group. Maternal and child undernutrition: Consequences for adult health and human capital. Lancet. 2008; 371(9609): 340–57.

27. Adair LS, Martorell R, Stein AD, Hallal PC, Sachdev HS, Prabhakaran D, Wills AK, Norris SA, Dahly DL, Lee NR, Victora CG. Size at birth, weight gain in infancy and childhood, and adult blood pressure in 5 low-and middle-income-country cohorts: When does weight gain matter? Am J Clin Nutr. 2009; 89(5): 1383–92

28. Stein AD, Wang M, Martorell R, Norris SA, Adair LS, Bas I, Sachdev HS, Bhargava SK, Fall CHD, Gigante DP, Victora CG on behalf of the COHORTS group. Growth patterns in early childhood and final attained stature: Data from five birth cohorts from low and middle income countries. Am J Hum Biol. 2010; 22(3): 353–59.

29. Martorell R, Horta BL, Adair LS, Stein AD, Richter L, Fall CH, Bhargava SK, Biswas SK, Perez L, Barros FC, Victora CG; Consortium on Health Orientated Research in Transitional Societies Group (includes Sachdev HS). Weight gain in the first two years of life is an important predictor of schooling outcomes in pooled analyses from five birth cohorts from low- and middle-income group countries. J Nutr. 2010; 140(2): 348–54.

30. Ramakrishnan L, Fall CH, Sachdev HS, Osmond C, Prabhakaran D, Biswas SD, Tandon N, Ramji S, Reddy KS, Barker DJ, Bhargava SK. Childhood body mass index and adult pro-inflammatory and pro-thrombotic risk factors: Data from the New Delhi birth cohort. Int J Epidemiol. 2011; 40(1): 102–11.

31. Fall CH, Borja JB, Osmond C, Richter L, Bhargava SK, Martorell R, Stein AD, Barros FC, Victora CG; COHORTS group. Infant-feeding patterns and cardiovascular risk factors in young adulthood: Data from five cohorts in low- and middle-income countries. Int J Epidemiol. 2011; 40(1): 47–62.

32. Paul VK, Sachdev HS, Mavalankar D, Ramachandran P, Jeeva Sankar M, Bhandari N, Sreenivas V, Sundararaman T, Govil D, Osrin D, Kirkwood B. Reproductive health, and child health and nutrition in India: Meeting the challenge. Lancet. 2011; 377(9762): 332–49

33. Huffman MD, Prabhakaran D, Osmond C, Fall CH, Tandon N, Lakshmy R, Ramji S, Khalil A, Gera T, Prabhakaran P, Biswas SK,Reddy KS, Bhargava SK, Sachdev HS; New Delhi Birth Cohort. Incidence of cardiovascular risk factors in an Indian urban cohort results from the New Delhi birth cohort. J Am Coll Cardiol. 2011; 57(17): 1765–74.

34. Ramakrishnan L, Sachdev HS, Sharma M, Abraham R, Prakash S, Gupta D, Singh Y, Bhaskar S, Sinha S, Chandak GR, Reddy KS, Bhargava S. Relationship of APOA5, PPARγ and HL gene variants with serial changes in childhood body mass index and coronary artery disease risk factors in young adulthood. Lipids Health Dis. 2011; 10(1): 68.

35. Finucane MM, Stevens GA, Cowan MJ, Danaei G, Lin JK, Paciorek CJ, Singh GM, Gutierrez HR, Lu Y, Bahalim AN, Farzadfar F, Riley LM, Ezzati M; Global Burden of Metabolic Risk Factors of Chronic Diseases Collaborating Group (Body Mass Index) (includes Sachdev HS). National, regional, and global trends in bodymass index since 1980: Systematic analysis of health examination surveys and epidemiological studies with 960 country-years and 9.1 million participants. Lancet. 2011; 377(9765): 557–67.

36. Danaei G, Finucane MM, Lu Y, Singh GM, Cowan MJ, Paciorek CJ, Lin JK, Farzadfar F, Khang YH, Stevens GA, Rao M, Ali MK, Riley LM, Robinson CA, Ezzati M; Global Burden of Metabolic Risk Factors of Chronic Diseases Collaborating Group (Blood Glucose). National, regional, and global trends in fasting plasma glucose and

diabetes prevalence since 1980: Systematic analysis of health examination surveys and epidemiological studies with 370 country-years and 2.7 million participants. Lancet. 2011; 378(9785): 31–40.

37. Richter LM, Victora CG, Hallal PC, Adair LS, Bhargava SK, Fall CH, Lee N, Martorell R, Norris SA, Sachdev HS, Stein AD; COHORTS Group. Cohort profile: The consortium of health-orientated research in transitioning societies. Int J Epidemiol. 2012; 41(3): 621–26.

38. Norris SA, Osmond C, Gigante D, Kuzawa CW, Ramakrishnan L, Lee NR, Ramirez-Zea M, Richter LM, Stein AD, Tandon N, Fall CH; COHORTS Group (includes Sachdev HS). Size at birth, weight gain in infancy and childhood, and adult diabetes risk in five low- or middle-income country birth cohorts. Diabetes Care. 2012; 35(1): 72–79.

39. Kuzawa CW, Hallal PC, Adair L, Bhargava SK, Fall CH, Lee N, Norris SA, Osmond C, Ramirez-Zea M, Sachdev HS, Stein AD, Victora CG; COHORTS Group. Birth weight, postnatal weight gain, and adult body composition in five low and middle income countries. Am J Hum Biol 2012; 24(1): 5–13.

40. Tandon N, Fall CH, Osmond C, Sachdev HP, Prabhakaran D, Ramakrishnan L, Dey Biswas SK, Ramji S, Khalil A, Gera T, Reddy KS, Barker DJ, Cooper C, Bhargava SK. Growth from birth to adulthood and peak bone mass and density data from the New Delhi Birth Cohort. Osteoporos Int 2012; 23(10): 2447–59.

41. Schillaci MA, Sachdev HP, Bhargava SK. Technical note: Comparison of the Maresh reference data with the WHO international standard for normal growth in healthy children. Am J Phys Anthropol. 2012; 147(3): 493–98.

42. Khalil A, Huffman MD, Prabhakaran D, Osmond C, Fall CHD, Tandon N, Lakshmy R, Prabhakaran P, Dey Biswas SK, Ramji S, Sachdev HS, Bhargava SK; New Delhi Birth Cohort. Predictors of carotid intima-media thickness and carotid plaque in young Indian adults: The New Delhi Birth Cohort. Int J Cardiol. 2012; 167(4): 1322–28.

43. Addo OY, Stein AD, Fall CH, Gigante DP, Guntupalli AM, Horta BL, Kuzawa CW, Lee N, Norris SA, Prabhakaran P, Richter LM, Sachdev HS, Martorell R; Consortium on Health Orientated Research in Transitional Societies (COHORTS) Group. Maternal Height and Child Growth Patterns. J Pediatr. 2013; 163(2): 549–54.

44. Danaei G, Singh GM, Paciorek CJ, Lin JK, Cowan MJ, Finucane MM, Farzadfar F, Stevens GA, Riley LM, Lu Y, Rao M, Ezzati M; Global Burden of Metabolic Risk Factors of Chronic Diseases Collaborating Group (includes Sachdev HS). The global cardiovascular risk transition: Associations of four metabolic risk factors with national income, urbanization, and Western diet in 1980 and 2008. Circulation. 2013; 127(14): 1493–502.

45. Adair LS, Fall CHD, Osmond C, Stein AD, Martorell R, Ramirez-Zea M, Sachdev HS, Dahly DL, Bas I, Norris SA, Micklesfield L, Hallal P, Victora CG, for the COHORTS group. Associations of linear growth and relative weight gain during early life with adult health and human capital in countries of low and middle income: Findings from five birth cohort studies. Lancet. 2013; 382(9891): 525–34.

46. Horta BL, Bas A, Bhargava SK, Fall CH, Feranil A, de Kadt J, Martorell R, Richter LM, Stein AD, Victora CG; COHORTS group (includes Sachdev HS). Infant feeding and school attainment in five cohorts from low- and middle-income countries. PLoS One. 2013; 8(8): e71548.

47. The Global Burden of Metabolic Risk Factors for Chronic Diseases Collaboration (includes Sachdev HS). Cardiovascular disease, chronic kidney disease, and diabetes mortality burden of cardiometabolic risk factors from 1980 to 2010: A comparative risk assessment. Lancet Diabetes Endocrinol. Early Online Publication; 17 May 2014. doi:10.1016/S2213-8587(14)70102-0

48. Lundeen EA, Stein AD, Adair LS, Behrman JR, Bhargava SK, Dearden KA, Gigante D, Norris SA, Richter LM, Fall CH, Martorell R, Sachdev HS, Victora CG on behalf of the COHORTS investigators. Height-for-age z scores increase despite increasing height deficits among children in 5 developing countries. Am J Clin Nutr. 2014; 9 July; 100(3): 821–25. pii: ajcn.084368. [Epub ahead of print]

49. Addo OY, Stein AD, Fall CHD, Gigante DP, Guntupalli AM, Horta BL, Kuzawa CW, Lee N, Norris SA, Osmond C, Prabhakaran P, Richter LM, Sachdev HPS, Martorell R. Parental childhood growth and offspring birthweight: Pooled analyses from four birth cohorts in low and middle income countries. Am J Hum Biol. 2015; 27: 99–105.

50. Fall CH, Sachdev HS, Osmond C, Restrepo-Mendez MC, Victora C, Martorell R, Stein AD, Sinha S, Tandon N, Adair L, Bas I, Norris S, Richter LM; COHORTS investigators. Association between

maternal age at childbirth and child and adult outcomes in the offspring: A prospective study in five low-income and middle-income countries (COHORTS collaboration). Lancet Glob Health. 2015; 31 July; 3(7): e366–77. pii: S2214-109X(15)00038-8. doi: 10.1016/S2214-109X(15)00038-8. [Epub ahead of print].

51. NCD Risk Factor Collaboration (NCD-RisC; includes Bhargava SK, Sachdev HS, Fall CHD, Osmond C). Effects of diabetes definition on global surveillance of diabetes prevalence and diagnosis: A pooled analysis of 96 population-based studies with 331 288 participants. Lancet Diabetes Endocrinol. 2015; 19 June. pii: S2213-8587(15)00129-1. doi: 10.1016/S2213-8587(15)00129-1. [Epub ahead of print] PubMed PMID: 26109024.

52. Huffman MD, Khalil A, Osmond C, Fall CH, Tandon N, Lakshmy R, Ramji S, Gera T, Prabhakaran P, Dey Biswas SK, Reddy KS, Bhargava SK, Sachdev HS, Prabhakaran D; New Delhi Birth Cohort. Association between anthropometry, cardiometabolic risk factors, & early life factors & adult measures of endothelial function: Results from the New Delhi Birth Cohort. Indian J Med Res. 2015; (Dec); 142(6): 690–98.

53. NCD Risk Factor Collaboration (NCD-RisC includes Sachdev HS, Bhargava SK, Fall CHD, Osmond CO). Trends in adult bodymass index in 200 countries from 1975 to 2014: A pooled analysis of 1698 population-based measurement studies with 19.2 million participants. Lancet. 2016; 387: 1377–96.

54. NCD Risk Factor Collaboration (NCD-RisC includes Sachdev HS, Bhargava SK, Fall CHD, Osmond CO). Worldwide trends in diabetes since 1980: A pooled analysis of 751 population-based studies with 4·4 million participants. Lancet. 2016; 387(10027): 1513–30.

55. NCD Risk Factor Collaboration (NCD-RisC includes Sachdev HS, Bhargava SK, Fall CHD, Osmond CO). A century of trends in adult human height. eLife. 2016; 5: e13410. DOI: 10.7554/eLife.13410.

56. Fall CHD, Osmond C, Haazen DS, Sachdev HS, Victora C, Martorell R, Stein AD, Adair L, Norris S, Richter LM, COHORTS Group. Disadvantages of having an adolescent mother. Lancet Glob Health. 2016; 4(11): e787–e788; DOI: http://dx.doi.org/10.1016/ S2214-109X(16)30263-7.

57. Sinha S, Aggarwal AR, Osmond C, Fall CH, Bhargava SK, Sachdev HS. Maternal age at childbirth and perinatal and under five mortality in a prospective birth cohort from Delhi. Indian Pediatr. 2016; 8 October; 53(10): 871–77.

58. NCD Risk Factor Collaboration (NCD-RisC includes Sachdev HS, Bhargava SK, Fall CHD, Osmond CO). Worldwide trends in blood pressure from 1975 to 2015: A pooled analysis of 1479 population-based measurement studies with 19·1 million participants. Lancet 2016; 15 November. http://dx.doi.org/10.1016/ S0140-6736(16)31919-5. Published Online 15 November 2016.

59. Sinha S, Aggarwal AR, Osmond C, Hd Fall C, Bhargava SK, Sachdev HS. Intergenerational Change in Anthropometric Indices of children and their Predictors in New Delhi Birth Cohort. Indian Pediatr. 2016; 5 December; 54: 185–92. pii: S097475591600033. [Epub ahead of print] PubMed PMID: 28031545.

# Bibliography

[1] Drillien CM. A longitudinal study of the growth and development of prematurely and maturely born children. Part I and II. Arch Dis Child. 1958; 33: 10 and 423.

[2] Nadkarni MG. An analysis of premature births at a public maternity hospital in Bombay. Indian J Child Hlth. 1960; 9: 239.

[3] Dann M, Levine SZ, Elizabek VN A long-term follow-up study of small premature infants. Pediatr. 1964; 33: 945–55.

[4] Harper PA, Wiener, G. Sequelae of low birth weight. Ann Rev Med. 1965; 16: 405–18.

[5] Bhargava V, Ghosh S, Bhargava SK: Survival, growth and development pattern in low birth weight babies in first year. Indian Pediatr. 1970; 7: 139.

[6] Bhakoo ON, Narang A, Kulkarni KN, Patil AS, Banerjee CK, Walia BNS. Neonatal morbidity and mortality in hospital born babies. Indian Pediatr. 1975; 12: 443–50.

[7] Bhargava SK, Bhargava V, Taneja S, Ghosh S Birth weight, gestational age and growth pattern in babies with a birth weight of 2000g or less. Indian Pediatr. 1971; 8: 736.

[8] Bhatia BD, Mathur NB, Chaturvedi P, Dubey AP. Neonatal mortality pattern in a rural based medical college hospital. Indian J. Pediatr. 1984; 51: 309.

[9] Bhargava SK. A study of the relationship of etiological factors, growth and development pattern to birth weight and gestational age in babies with a birth weight of 2000 gm or less. Final Report of an Indian Council of Medical Research Enquiry. 1978.

[10] Singh M, Tripathy K, Arya LS. Birth weight, gestational age correlates of neonatal mortality. Indian J. Pediatr. 1982; 49: 511.

[11] Bhargava SK, Kumari S, Choudhury P. Out-come of low birth weight infants. Acta Pediatr Scand. 1984; 73: 406–07.

[12] Bhatia BD, Mathur NB, Chaturvedi P, Dubey AP. Neonatal mortality pattern in a rural based medical college hospital. Indian J. Pediatr. 1984; 51: 309.

[13] Hack M, Klein NK, Taylor, HG. Long-term developmental outcomes of low birth weight infants. Future Child. 1995; 5: 176–96.

[14] Saigal S, Doyle LW. An overview of mortality and sequelae of preterm birth from infancy to adulthood. Lancet. 2008; 371: 261–69.

[15] Aarnoudse-Moens CSH, Weisglas-Kuperus N, van Goudoever JB, Oosterlaan J. Meta-analysis of neurobehavioral outcomes in very preterm and/or very low birth weight children. Pediatr. 2009; 124(2): 261–69.

[16] Barker DJP, Hales CN, Fall CHD, Osmond C, Phipps K, Clark PMC. Type 2 (non-insulin-dependent) diabetes mellitus, hypertension and hyperlipidemia (syndrome X): Relation to reduced foetal growth. Diabetologia.1993; 36: 62–67.

[17] Barker DJ. Fetal origins of coronary heart disease. BMJ. 1995; 311(6998): 171–74.

[18] Curhan GC, Willett WC, Rimm EB, Spiegelman D, Ascherio AL, Stampfer MJ. Birth weight and adult hypertension, diabetes mellitus, and obesity in US men. BMI. 1996; 94(12): 3246–50.

[19] Frankel S, Elwood P, Swertham P, Yarnell J, Smith ED. Birth weight, body mass index and incident coronary heart disease. Lancet. 1996; 348: 1478–80.

[20] Bhargava SK, Sachdev HS, Caroline HD, Fall DM, Osmond C, Lakshmy R, Barker DJP, Biswas SK, Ramji S, Prabhakaran D, Reddy KS. Relation of serial changes in childhood body-mass index to impaired glucose tolerance in young adulthood. The N Engl J Med. 2004; 350(9): 865–75.

[21] Ghosh S, Beri S. Standard of prematurity for North Indian babies. The Indian J Child Health. 1962; (May); 11: 210–15.

[22] Ghosh S, Daga S. Comparison of gestational age and weight as standards of prematurity. J Peadiatr. 1967; 71: 173–75.

[23] Yerushalmy J. The classification of newborn infants by birth weight and gestational age. J Paediatr. 1967; 71: 164–72.

[24] Bataglia FC, Lubcheno LO. A practical classification of newborn infants by weight and gestational age. J of Paediatr. 1967; 71: 159–63.

[25] Das NC, Dasgupta A. Fertility in India-trends differentials, implications. Indian J Public Health. 1974; 18: 138.

[26] Mitra A. Age at marriage. Paper presented in Second Annual Conference of Indian Association for the study population. Institute for Social and Economic Change. Bangalore, 1976.

[27] Martin JA, Brady MPH, Hamilton E, et al. Division of vital statistics, births: Final data for 2013. Natl Vital Stat Rep. 2015; 64(1): 1–65.

[28] Kulkarni, PM. Towards an explanation of India's fertility transition. George Simmons Memorial Lecture delivered at the 33rd Annual Conference of Indian Association for the Study of Population (IASP), Lucknow; November 11–13, 2011.

[29] Kaur, H. Impact of income and education on fertility. J Fam Welf. 2000; 46(1): 70–76.

[30] Ghosh S, Bhargava SK, Madhavan S, Taskar AD, Bhargava V, and Nigam SK. Interauterine growth of North Indian babies. Paediatr. 1971; 47: 826.

[31] Papageorghiou AT, Ohuma EO, Altman DG, et al. International standard for fetal growth based on serial ultrasound measurement: The fetal growth 869-longitudinal study of the INTERGROWTH-21st project. Lancet. 2014; 384; 869–79. doi: 10.1016/S0140–6736(14)61490–2.

[32] Villar J, Ismai LC, Victora CG. International standards for newborn weight, length, and head circumference by gestational age and sex: The newborn cross-sectional study of the INTERGROWTH-21st project. Lancet. 2014; 384(9946): 857–68. doi: 10.1016/S0140–6736(14)60932–6

[33] WHO. Expert group on prematurity: Final report. Technical Report Series No 27: 1950.

[34] Lubchenco LO, Hansman C, Boyd E. Intrauterine growth in length and head circumference as estimated from live births at gestational ages from 26 to 42 weeks. J Paediatr. 1966; 37: 403–08.

[35] Sachdev HPS. Low birth weight in South Asia. Int J Diabetes Dev Ctries. 2001: 21: 13–31.

[36] Chaudhari S, Otiv M, Khairnar B, Pandit A, Hoge M, Sayyad M. Pune low birth weight study: Growth from birth to adulthood. Indian Pediatr. 2012; 49: 727–32.

[37] Cruise MO. A longitudinal study of the growth of low birth weight infants: Velocity and distance growth. Paediatr. 1970; 51: 620.

[38] Bhargava SK, Bhargava V, Taneja S, Ghosh S. Birth weight, gestational age and growth pattern in babies with a birth weight of 2000 g or less. Indian Pediatr. 1971; 8: 736.

[39] Chaudhari S, Otiv M, Chitale A, Pandit A, Hoge M. Pune low birth weight study: Cognitive abilities and educational performance at twelve years. Indian Pediatr., 2004; 41: 121–28.

[40] Bhargava SK, Kumari S. Chaudhary P, et al. Longitudinal study of linear physical growth of infants with birth weight 1500g or less from birth to six years. Indian J Med Res. 1983; 78: 78–82.

[41] Bhargava SK, Kumari S, Chaudhary P, et al. Longitudinal study of linear physical growth in preterm infants from birth to six years. Indian. J Med Res. 1983; 78: 74–77.

[42] Bhargava SK, Kumari S, Chaudhary P, Butani R, Sachdev HPS. A longitudinal study of physical growth of small for date infants, from birth to six years. Nutr Res. 1985; 5: 707–13.

[43] Ranke MB, Vollmer B, Traunecker R, Wollman HA, Goelz RR, Seibolweiger K. Growth and development are similar in VLBW children born appropriate and small for gestational age: An interim report of 97 preschool children. J Pediatr Endocrinol Metab. 1997; 20: 1017–26.

[44] Paz I, Seidman DS, Danon YL, Laor A, Stevenson DK, Gale R. Are children born small for gestational age at increased risk of short stature? Am J Dis Child Pediatr Res. 1993; 147: 337–39.

[45] Beargie RA. Growth and development of small for dates new born. PCNA, 1970; 15: 159.

[46] Bhargava S, Ghosh S, and Lall UB. A study of low birth weight infants in an urban community. Health Popul Perspect Issues.1979; 2(1): 54–65.

[47] Ghosh S, Gidwani S, Mittal SK, Verma RK. Socio-cultural factors affecting breast feeding practices in an urban community. Indian Pediatr. 1976; 13(11): 827–32.

[48] Countdown to 2015. A decade of tracking progress for maternal, newborn and child Survival. Geneva, WHO and UNICEF: The 2015 Report, 110–11.

[49] http://www.indexmundi.com/facts/india/mortality-rate under five

[50] http://www.indexmundi.com/facts/india/mortality-rate neonatal

[51] Ghosh S, Ramanujacharyulu TK, Hooja V, Madhavan S. Mortality pattern in an urban birth cohort. Indian J Med Res. 1979; 69: 616–23.

[52] Report of National Neonatal Perinatal Database (NNPD) 2002–2003. Available from: http://www.newbornwhocc.org/nnpo.html. Accessed 20 January 2014.

[53] Hooja V, Madhavan S, Ahmad SH, Ghosh S. Outcome and survival of a birth cohort in a community of South Delhi: Preliminary report of prospective study. Indian Pediatr. 1972; 9: 495–505.

[54] Bhargava SK, Banerjee SK, Chaudhary P, Kumari S. A longitudinal study of morbidity and mortality pattern from birth to six years of age in infants of varying birth weight, Indian Pediatr. 1979; 16: 967–73.

[55] Kulshreshta R, Nath, LM, Upadhaya P. Congenital malformations in live born infants in rural community. Indian Pediatr, 1983; 20; 45–48. Report of the National Neonatal Perinatal.

[56] Database. Report 2002–2003. NNPD Network. 2005.

[57] Ghosh S, Bhargava SK, Butani R. Congenital malformations in a longitudinally studied birth cohort in an urban community. Indian J Med Res. 1985; 82: 427–33.

[58] Hooja V, Ghosh S, Mittal SK, Verma RK. Immunization status in an urban community. Indian Pediatr. 1976; 13: 747–50.

[59] Indian Council of Medical Research. Growth and physical development of Indian infants and children. Technical Report Series No. 18, 1989.

[60] Agarwal DK, Agarwal KN. Physical growth of Indian affluent children (Birth–6 years). Indian Pediatr. 1994; 31: 377–413.

[61] Agarwal DK, Agarwal KN, Upadhyay SK, Mittal R, Prakash R, Rai S. Physical and sexual growth pattern of affluent Indian children from 5–18 years of age. Indian Pediatr. 1992; 29: 1203–82.

[62] WHO Multicentre Growth Reference Study Group. Assessment of differences in linear growth among populations in the WHO Multicentre Growth Reference Study. Acta Paediatrica. Supplementum 2006; 450: 56–65.

[63] Khadilkar V, Yadav S, Agarwal K, Tamboli S, Banerjee M, Cherian A, et al. Revised IAP growth charts for height, weight and body mass index for 5 to 18 year old Indian children. Indian Pediatr. 2015, 52: 47–55.

[64] Vijayaraghavan K, Sastry JG, Jindal IB. Growth performance of well-to-do Hyderabad children: A follow-up study. Indian J Med Res. 1974; 62: 117–24.

[65] Kaul, S. Growth in three anthropometric measures in Kashmiri Pandit school going boys with some observations on the efficiency of mixed longitudinal analysis of human growth. Indian J. Med. Res. 1975; 63: 590–96.

[66] Seth V, Ghai OP, Sugathan TN. Velocity of growth in schoolchildren. Indian Pediatr. 1972; 9: 746–50.

[67] Terman, LM, Merrill MA. The Stanford-Binet intelligence scale: Manual for third revision from LM. Norms Edition. Boston: Houghton Mifflin; 1973.

[68] Rao A, Anandalakshmy S. Patterns of linguistic communication in preschool children of two socio economic status levels. Paper read at the Institute of Advanced Study, Simla, in the Seminar on Language and Culture in 1973. Available from: http://ijsw.tiss.edu/greenstone/collect/ijsw/index/assoc/HASHc762/0d1f164b.dir/doc.pdf).

[69] Kapani V. A Longitudinal study of Survival and outcome of a Birth Cohort Report. 1995.

[70] WHO. Growth reference 5–19 years. http://www.who.int/growthref/who 2007_bmi_for_age/en/index.html

[71] Shakir A, Morley D. Letter measuring malnutrition. Lancet. 1974; 20 April: 1(7860): 758–59.

[72] Richter LM, Victora CG, Hallal PC, Adair LS, Bhargava SK, Fall CH, Lee N, Martorell R, Norris SA, Sachdev HS, et al. COHORTS Group. Cohort profile: The consortium of health-orientated research in transitioning societies. Int J Epidemiol. 2012; 41: 621–26.

[73] Bhargava SK, Sachdev HS, Fall CHD, Osmond C, Lakshmy R, Barker DJP, Biswas SKD, Ramji S, Prabhakaran D, Reddy KS. Relation of serial changes in childhood body-mass index to impaired glucose tolerance in young adulthood. N Engl J Med. 2004; 350: 865–75.

[74] Norris SA, Osmond C, Gigante D, Kuzawa CW, Ramakrishnan L, Lee NR, Ramirez-Zea M, Richter LM, Stein AD, Tandon N, Fall CH, COHORTS Group (includes Sachdev HS). Size at birth, weight gain in infancy and childhood, and adult diabetes risk in five low- or middle-income country birth cohorts. Diabetes Care. 2012; 35: 72–79.

[75] Whincup PH, Kaye SJ, Owen CG, Huxley R, Cook DG, Anazawa S, Barrett-Connor E, Bhargava SK, Birgisdottir BE, Carlsson S, de Rooij SR, Dyck RF, Eriksson JG, Falkner B, Fall C, Forsén T, Grill V, Gudnason V, Hulman S, Hyppönen E, Jeffreys M, Lawlor DA, Leon DA, Minami J, Mishra G, Osmond C, Power C, Rich-Edwards JW, Roseboom TJ, Sachdev HS, Syddall H, Thorsdottir I, Vanhala M, Wadsworth M, Yarbrough DE. Birth weight and risk of type 2 diabetes. JAMA. 2008; 300: 2886–97.

[76] Sachdev HS, Osmond C, Fall CH, Lakshmy R, Ramji S, Dey Biswas S, Prabhakaran D, Tandon N, Reddy KS, Barker DJP, Bhargava SK. Predicting adult metabolic syndrome from childhood body mass index: Follow-up of the New Delhi birth cohort. Arch Dis Child. 2009; 94(10): 768–74.

[77] Fall CH, Sachdev HS, Osmond C, Lakshmy R, Dey Biswas S, Prabhakaran D, Tandon N, Ramji S, Reddy KS, Barker DJ, Bhargava SK. Adult metabolic syndrome and impaired glucose tolerance are associated with different patterns of body mass index gain during infancy; Data from the New Delhi birth cohort. Diabetes Care. 2008; 31(12): 2349–56.

[78] Sachdev HS, Fall CHD, Osmond C, Lakshmy R, Biswas SKD, Leary SD, Reddy KS, Barker DJP, Bhargava SK. Anthropometric indicators of body composition in young adults: Relation to size at birth and serial measurements of body mass index in childhood in the New Delhi birth cohort. Am J Clin Nutr. 2005; 82: 456–66.

[79] Kuzawa CW, Hallal PC, Adair L, Bhargava SK, Fall CH, Lee N, Norris SA, Osmond C, Ramirez-Zea M, Sachdev HS, Stein AD, Victora CG, COHORTS Group. Birth weight, postnatal weight gain, and adult body composition in five low and middle income countries. Am J Hum Biol. 2012; 24: 5–13.

[80] Tandon N, Fall CH, Osmond C, Sachdev HP, Prabhakaran D, Ramakrishnan L, Dey Biswas SK, Ramji S, Khalil A, Gera T, Reddy KS, Barker DJ, Cooper C, Bhargava SK. Growth from birth to adulthood and peak bone mass and density data from the New Delhi Birth Cohort. Osteoporos Int. 2012; 23(10): 2447–59.

[81] Schillaci MA, Sachdev HP, Bhargava SK. Technical note: Comparison of the Maresh reference data with the WHO international standard for normal growth in healthy children. Am J Phys Anthropol. 2012; 147(3): 493–98.

[82] Lakshmy R, Fall CHD, Sachdev HS, Osmond C, Prabhakaran D, Biswas SD, Tandon N, Ramji S, Reddy KS, Barker DJP, Bhargava SK. Childhood body mass index and adult pro-inflammatory and pro-thrombotic risk factors: Data from the New Delhi birth cohort. Int J Epidemiol. 2011; 40(1): 102–11.

[83] Huffman MD, Prabhakaran D, Osmond C, Fall CHD, Tandon N, Lakshmy R, Ramji S, Khalil A, Gera T, Prabhakaran P, Dey Biswas SK, Reddy KS, Bhargava SK, Sachdev HS on behalf of New Delhi Birth Cohort. Incidence of cardiovascular risk factors in an Indian urban cohort: Results from the New Delhi Birth Cohort. J Amer Coll Cardiol. 2011; 57: 1765–74.

[84] Khalil A, Huffman MD, Prabhakaran D, Osmond C, Fall CHD, Tandon N, Lakshmy R,Prabhakaran P, Dey Biswas SK, Ramji S, Sachdev HS, Bhargava SK on behalf of the New Delhi Birth Cohort. Predictors of carotid intima-media thickness and carotid plaque in young Indian adults: The New Delhi Birth Cohort. Int J Cardiol. 2012; 167(4): 1322–28.

[85] Fall CH, Borja JB, Osmond C, Richter L, Bhargava SK, Martorell R, Stein AD, Barros FC, Victora CG, COHORTS group. Infant-feeding patterns and

cardiovascular risk factors in young adulthood: Data from five cohorts in low- and middle-income countries. Int J Epidemiol. 2011; 40(1): 47–62.

[86] Horta BL, Bas A, Bhargava SK, Fall CH, Feranil A, de Kadt J, Martorell R, Richter LM, Stein AD, Victora CG, COHORTS group (includes Sachdev HS). Infant feeding and school attainment in five cohorts from low- and middle-income countries. PLoS One. 2013; 20 August; 8(8): e71548. doi: 10.1371/journal.pone.0071548.

[87] Stein AD, Wang M, Martorell R, Norris SA, Adair LS, Bas I, Sachdev HS, Bhargava SK, Fall CHD, Gigante DP, Victora CG on behalf of the COHORTS group. Growth patterns in early childhood and final attained stature: Data from five birth cohorts from low and middle income countries. Am J Human Biol. 2010; 22: 353–59.

[88] Martorell R, Horta BL, Adair LS, Stein AD, Richter L, Fall CHD, Bhargava SK, Dey Biswas SK, Perez L, Barros FC, Victora CG, Consortium on Health Orientated Research in Transitioning Societies Group (includes Sachdev HS). Weight gain in the first two years of life is an important predictor of schooling outcomes in pooled analyses from five birth cohorts from low- and middle-income group countries. J Nutr. 2010; 140: 348–54.

[89] Adair LS, Fall CH, Osmond CStein AD, Martorell R, Ramirez-Zea M, Sachdev HP, Dahly DL, Bas I, Norris SA, Micklesfield L, Hallal P, Victora CG, COHORTS group. Associations of linear growth and relative weight gain during early life with adult health and human capital in countries of low and middle income: Findings from five birth cohort studies. Lancet. 2013; 382(9891): 525–34.

[90] Stein AD, Barros FC, Bhargava SK, Hao W, Horta BL, Lee N, Kuzawa CW, Martorell R, Ramji S, Stein A, Richter L, Consortium of Health-Orientated Research in Transitioning Societies (COHORTS) investigators (includes Sachdev HS). Birth status, child growth, and adult outcomes in low- and middle-income countries. J Pediatr. 2013; 163(6): 1740–46.

[91] Addo OY, Stein AD, Fall CHD, Gigante DP, Guntupalli AM, Horta BL, Kuzawa CW, Lee N, Norris SA, Osmond C, Prabhakaran P, Richter LM, Sachdev HPS, Martorell R, on behalf of the COHORTS Group. Parental childhood growth and offspring birthweight: Pooled analyses from four birth cohorts in low and middle income countries. Am. J. Hum Biol. 2015; 27: 99–105.

[92] Addo OY, Stein AD, Fall CH, Gigante DP, Guntupalli AM, Horta BL, Kuzawa CW, Lee N, Norris SA, Prabhakaran P, Richter LM, Sachdev HS, Martorell R, Consortium on Health Orientated Research in Transitional Societies (COHORTS) group. Maternal height and child growth patterns. J Pediatr. 2013; 163(2): 549–54.

[93] Victora CG, Adair L, Fall C, Hallal PC, Martorell R, Richter L, Sachdev HS, Maternal and Child Undernutrition Study Group. Maternal and child undernutrition: Consequences for adult health and human capital. Lancet. 2008; 371(9609): 340–57.

[94] Fall CHD, Sachdev HS, Osmond C, Restrepo-Mendez MC, Victora C, Martorell R, et al. Association between maternal age at childbirth and child and adult outcomes in the offspring: A prospective study in five low-income and middle-income countries (COHORTS collaboration). Lancet Glob Health. 2015; 1 July: 3(7): e366–e377.

[95] Ramakrishnan L, Sachdev HS, Sharma M, Abraham R, Prakash S, Gupta D, Singh Y, Bhaskar S, Sinha S, Chandak GR, Reddy KS, Bhargava S. Relationship of APOA5, PPAR gamma and HL gene variants with serial changes in childhood body mass index and coronary artery disease risk factors in young adulthood. Lipids Health Dis. 2011; 8 May: 10(1): 68. [doi:10.1186/1476–511X-10–68].

# Index

abortions, 27, 39, 52
Adair, L., 145
adolescence, 2, 89, 106, 172, 175, 185, 199, 237, 255
  body composition, 173
  body growth during, 107
  cardiovascular risk among, 205
adult anthropometry, 180
adult body composition, 174
adult diseases, 173, 174, 237–239
adult follow-up, 28
adult health, 4, 145, 180, 207, 240
adult human capital, 180
adult metabolic syndrome, 171
adult stature, 165, 180, 183
  growth pattern in, 179
  human capital development, assessment of, 256
  income generation, 240
adulthood, 1, 2, 3, 7, 76, 82, 89, 108, 144, 165, 167, 174, 182, 218, 251, 260
age
  at first pregnancy, 37–38
  at marriage, 19, 35
All India Institute of Medical Sciences, 147
antenatal care, 50
anthropometric indicators, 173, 174
anthropometry, 130
  intergenerational changes in, 208
  measurements, 194
APOA, 5, 185

appropriate for gestation age (AGA), 68, 70, 83, 181, 251
areal bone mineral density (aBMD), 175
Attention Deficit Hyperactive Disorder, 207
attrition or loss to follow-up, 259
  expired, 212
  in different phases of NDBC, 212–216
  permanent loss cases, 211
  reasons for, 216–217
  refusal, 212
  reluctant, 212
  shifted or moved out or moved in cases, 211
  temporary loss, 212

Barker, David, 85
Barker's Hypothesis of "Foetal Origin of Adult Disease", 3
BCG vaccine, 99
Bhargava, Santosh K., 9, 10, 145, 249
Bill and Mellinda Gates Foundation, 145
Birth Cohort study
  based on large community cohort, 2
  data collection from urban community, 3
  establishment of, 2
birth of cohorts, 53, 250
birth size, 180

telomere length in adulthood,
relationship to, 187
Birth to Twenty Study (BT, 20), South
Africa, 145
birth weight, 3, 60, 170, 174
and gestation period, 70
area of concern, 7
genetic determinants of, 187
importance of, 7
neonatal mortality among low
birth weight groups, 73
body composition, 2, 3, 89, 144, 146,
171, 173, 174, 180, 185, 259,
237, 239
body growth, 3, 175, 171, 172
body growth measurements
analysis of, 105
from 11 to 19 years or adolescence, 107
from 6 to 10 years, 107
from birth to five years, 107
interpretation of parameters, 105,
106
methods of, 103
sampling study, 103
techniques, 103
body growth
of preterm babies, 80
small gestation period impact on,
84
body mass index (BMI), 3, 167
and metabolic syndrome, 171
childhood, 171, 186
in infants, childhood and adolescence, higher, 174
prevalence in F1 and F2 generations, 208
body metabolism, 89
bone density, 144, 175, 255
bone mineral content (BMC), 144,
175
breastfeeding, 8, 27, 145, 184, 234
benefits of, 177, 178
practices in Cohort, 93
till 6 months of age, 134

British Heart Foundation, 144, 253

caesarean, 52
cardiovascular diseases, 8, 144, 255,
175–178
Cebu Longitudinal Health and
Nutrition Survey (CEBU),
Philippines, 145
Center for Chronic Diseases Control,
147
Central Government Health Scheme
(CGHS), 11
Central Institute of Education (CIE),
85, 120
individual scale of intelligence,
121
child behaviour checklist (CBCL),
207
child mortality, 2, 93, 96, 229, 230,
233, 234, 250, 251, 261
child survival, 39, 230, 233, 251, 261
childhood, 2
growth, 237–239
immunization, 235
nutrition, 3, 252
preschool years, 4
telomere length in adulthood,
relationship to, 187
children follow-up, 27
children global assessment scale
(CGAS), 207
Christian Medical College, Vellore, 9
cognitive development (CD), 252
developmental assessment, 128
follow-up at 6 years, 122
methods of, 121
observations, 122
cognitive development assessment
scales, 235
cohabitation, 37, 250, 261
community participation, challenges to
and expectations of participants,
245
attrition and loss to follow-up, 245

congenital anomalies, definition of, 98
congenital malformations, 9, 22, 23, 26, 27, 76, 96, 99, 251
Consortium of Health Oriented Research in Transiting societies (COHORTS), 253
Cooke, Dorothy, 9
coronary artery disease (CAD), 185
coronary heart disease (CHD), 89

delayed cry (asphyxia), 8
Detecto type scales, 15
Developmental Origin of Health and Adult Disease, 3
diabetes, 3, 68, 92, 130, 165, 167, 199, 229, 238, 253, 254, 256
  in young Delhi, phenotypic characterization of, 186
  India as capital of, 1
  mellitus, 144
  risk among adult, 168–170
DPT vaccine, 99
dysglycemic disorder, 180

early childhood, 1, 23, 27, 106, 171, 173, 182, 199
  growth pattern in, 179
elder mothers, 184
ever-married women, 41, 249
  profile of, 34, 250
  registration of, 25

facility based baby delivery, 52
family planning, 25, 250
  factors influencing, 43
  in population, practice, 41
family welfare, NDBC focus on, 229, 230
first pregnancy, 73, 261
  age at marriage, 37, 38

Gessels Developmental scale, 120
gestation term or period
  definition of, 54

preterm babies, growth pattern, 80
small, impact on growth patterns, 84
gestational age or period, 11, 27, 54, 144, 228
Ghosh, Shanti, 8, 9, 69, 249
Gluckman, Peter, 144
Goel, P. P., 16

hard grip, 208
high birth weight children, 3
Hooja, V., 17
human capital, 4, 180
  development, 68, 89, 106, 145, 183, 236, 240
hypertension, 3, 130, 253, 256
hysterectomy, 25

immunization, 99, 100, 199, 233
impaired glucose tolerance, 144, 166, 167, 168
incremental growth
  definition of, 116
  of boys, 118
  of girls, 118
Indian Council of Medical Research (ICMR), 9, 15, 146
  Children Growth Study in 1956, 16
infant feeding
  and cardiovascular risk factors young adults, 178
  and school attainment, 178
infantometers, 14
infants, 70, 250
  follow-up, 27
  intrauterine growth retarded, 2
  low birth weight, 7
  mortality, 3, 96
  premature/preterm, 55, 130
  telomere length in adulthood, relationship to, 187

Institute of Central America and Panama Nutrition Trial (INCAP), Guatemala, 145
institutional base baby delivery, 52
intelligence quotient (IQ), 85
intergenerational change, 258
  birth weight, 208
  in anthropometry, 208
  in malnutrition status of NDBC, 196, 199
  low birth weight, 208
  on birth weight and low birth weight prevalence, 195
  study, influence of, 242, 243
International Obesity Task Force, 106
intrauterine growth, 71, 66
intrauterine growth retarded (IUGR), 68, 232
ischaemic heart disease, 3

Jain, A. P., 14

lactation, 18, 21, 27
lady health visitors (LHV), 18
large for gestation (LGA), 71, 251
last menstrual period (LMP), 26
late age pregnancies, 183
late childhood, 144, 145, 172, 173
Longitudinal Study of the Survival and Outcome of a Birth Cohort Project
  registration of ever married women, 25
  area selection, 13
  census, repeating of, 22
  components of study, planning for, 22
  defining objectives of study, 22, 23
  ever-married women, profile of, 35
  fertility assessment, 35
  methodology of, 24
  physical characteristics and housing, 32
  planning of study, 10

population characteristics, 32–34
population, selection of, 10–13
procurement of tools and equipment, 15
pro forma development, 14
project staff and administrative office, locating, 16
recruitment of staff, 18
schedules and pro forma of study, 21
staff training and standardization of techniques, 18–19
statistical and data management tools and equipment, 16
team, 10
low birth weight (LBW) children, 2, 60, 251
  causes of, 73
  chronic adult diseases, rise in number of, 92
  definition of, 8, 68
  health complications among, 68, 76
  historical perspective of, 68, 69
  life course of NDBC, 92
  long term consequences of, 85–89
  prevalence across globe, 69

malnutrition, 22, 107, 129
  form of, 130
  in under five children, 130
  intergenerational changes in status of, 196
Maresh Reference data, 175
marriage
  age at, 37
  consummation of, 37
married pregnant women, 21
Martorell, R., 145
maternal literacy, 100
Maulana Azad Medical College, 147
menopause, 19, 25, 34
menstruation, 18
  status, 25

metabolic syndrome, 3, 130, 165, 166, 170, 177, 208, 229
mid-upper arm circumference (MUAC), 252
morbidity(ies), 8, 89
  causes of, 76
  newborn, 71
  old age, 8
  sleep disorders due to, 205
Moriyama, I. M., 9, 249
mortality, 1, 8, 73
  causes of, 76
  infant, 96
  newborn, 94
  under-five, 96
multicentre growth reference study (MGRS) group, 175

National Centre for Health Statistics (NCHS), USA, 9, 10, 108, 249
New Delhi Birth Cohort (NDBC), 3, 7, 10, 25, 54, 69, 89, 165
  adult diseases, 168
  adult period, beginning of, 147
  adult phase, 253
  age independent measurement of undernutrition, 236
  assembling of, 140–142
  birth measurements, 61
  birth weight, 168
  challenges faced by, 259, 260
  characteristics of, 157
  child health, statistics on, 233–235
  child survival, health and disease, 251
  child undernutrition, 240–241
  childhood growth and human capital development, 240
  childhood, growth in, 168
  clinic activities, 152
  convenience of, 220
  current status of, 149
  depository of research, 231, 232

distribution and interpretation of, 220
expectation of members, 259, 260
feature of, 76–79
field clinics organization, 152
four generations of, 191
growth monitoring, health and disease, 239, 240
growth pattern of, 109
growth studies, 252
growth studies, contribution towards, 236
head circumference, 61
indifference and problems, 222, 223
interactive meetings with, 221
intergeneration studies, result of, 262
intrauterine growth, 67, 232
length of cohort infants, 61
life course of, 92
low birth weight, investigation of problems, 232, 233
malnutrition, study on problems of, 236
maternal size influence, 240, 241
morbidity, 97, 98
participation of members, 259–260
participation, challenges to, 221–222
phases of, 139
post-clinic activity, 155
pre-clinic activities, 152
pregnancy outcome, 230
research area, 256–257
research project, implication and impact of, 260–262
reviving of, 148
size at birth, 168
size at birth, factors influencing, 62
social and cultural changes, 161
socio economic and wealth status, 159

socio-cultural and environmental characteristics in adult phase, 254
spouses occupation, 158
strategies to enhance participation, 223–224
three generations, sleep disorders in, 201
trans-generation, 258
trans-generation studies, result of, 262
transition to adult phase, 253
trust of, 219–220
newborn, 53
  birth weight of, 61
  head circumference, 61
  infants, 8
  length of, 61
  mortality, 94–96
  mortality in, 95
non-pregnant married women, 19
noninsulin-dependent diabetes mellitus (NIDDM), 89
nutrition, 1, 8, 43, 62, 66, 92, 96, 99, 252
  assessment, 131
  disorders, 130
nutritional abundance, 1

obesity, 1, 3, 4, 92, 106, 129, 145, 173, 199, 201, 257
offspring birth weight, 181
overnutrition, 199, 252
overweight, 1, 3, 92, 105, 129, 166, 170, 173, 180, 199, 207, 243

parental childhood growth, 181
parental genotype, 186
parental influences on adult health
  maternal and child undernutrition, 182, 183
  maternal height and child growth patterns, 182
  teenage and late age pregnancies, impact of, 184

Pelotas Birth Cohort Study, Brazil, 145
PL 480 scheme, 9, 14
Polio vaccine, 99
population explosion, NDBC focus on, 229, 230
postnatal weight gain, 174
pre schooling, 121
pregnancy(ies)/pregnant women, 18, 250
  antenatal care, 50
  delivery of bay, 52
  follow-up, 49, 26–27
  loss, effect of, 2
  number in users and non-users, 43
  outcome, 27
  status, 38, 39
premature/preterm baby(ies), 8
  definition of, 54
  prevalence across globe, 55
public health and policies, NDBC focus on, 228–229
public health authorities in India, aware about health problems, 7
Public Health Foundation of India, 147
Public Health Nurse (PHN), 12, 14, 18, 26

Rao, K. S. Sunder, 9
Richter, L., 145

S. L. Jain Hospital, 147
Safdarjung Hospital, New Delhi, 11, 12, 13, 16, 27, 249
secondary amenorrhea, 25
Singh, Indra Pal, 14
single generation study, 4
Sitaram Bhartia Institute of Science and Research, 147
small for gestation age (SGA), 68, 70, 71, 85, 181, 251
small pox vaccine, 99
social quotient, 85

Society for Nutrition Education and
    Health Action (SNEHA), 144
spacing between birth, 41
sterilization of husband or wife, 25
still births, 52, 250
stunting, 179, 134
    prevalence in F1 and F2 genera-
        tions, 208

Taskar, A. D., 9
teenage marriages, 50
teenage pregnancies, 184
telomere length in adulthood, 187
term infants, 70, 74, 250
    definition of, 54
third generation children, 244, 259
third generation of NDBC
    and hard grip, 208
    behavioural problems in school
        going children, 207
    cardiovascular risk factors in F1
        and F2 adolescences, 205
    general profile, 205
    sleep disorders and morbidities,
        205–207
trans-generation, 257
    deterioration, 4
    sleep disorders in three generations
        of NDBC, 201
    study on sleep disorders, 243
triglycerides risk factor, 185

Type 2 Diabetes, 146, 170, 186

undernutrition, 2, 94, 97, 199, 252,
    131
    age independent measurements
        of, 136
underweight, 1, 105, 129, 131, 243,
    262
    prevalence in F1 and F2 genera-
        tions, 208
UNICEF, 15
upper mid arm circumference
    (UMAC), 131, 136
USAID, 15

Victora, C., 145

wasting, 131, 133
    decrease with increase in age, 92
    prevalence in F1 and F2 genera-
        tion, 208
weight gain
    during early life, 180
    in first two years of life, 179–180
    in infancy and childhood, 168–170
World Health Organization (WHO),
    8, 15
    Standard Growth charts, 108

Yerushalmy, Jacob, 9
young mothers, 184

# About the Author

**Santosh K. Bhargava** is a leading consultant in paediatrics and neonatology. He is a former National President of the Indian Academy of Paediatrics; Founder President, National Neonatology Forum, India; Professor and Head, Department of Paediatrics, University College of Medical Sciences and Safdarjung Hospital, New Delhi; Editor, Indian Paediatrics.

He has been a member of several prestigious committees, such as the World Health Organization; Ministry of Health and Family Welfare, National Children Board, Planning Commission, Government of India, and Indian Council of Medical Research.

Prof. Bhargava has been a recipient of several research grants from national and international organizations such as the Indian Council of Medical Research and Department of Biotechnology, Government of India; National Center for Health Statistics, USA; Bill Gates Foundation; British Heart Foundation and Wellcome Trust, UK. He has published over 200 research papers in national and international accredited peer-reviewed journals. His primary research focuses on child health, newborns and public health issues. His contributions have been recognized by numerous national and international awards.